Karen Nimmo, MSc, PGDipClinPsych, DipPhysEd, MNZCCP, is a registered clinical psychologist with a private practice in Wellington. She also works as a psychologist in high-performance sport and runs workshops in confidence, self-esteem and peak performance. Karen was first hooked by the mind–body connection during her physical education studies as a teenager at the University of Otago. She later pursued this fascination through her psychology studies at Victoria University. Between her spells at 'school', Karen was a journalist in New Zealand, Australia and the United Kingdom, and ran a communications/media consultancy for several years. Karen lives in Wellington with her husband Kev and two teenage daughters. Away from work, she invests fully in life's simple pleasures: good company, a few laughs and a glass of wine.

MY BUM LOOKS BRILLIANT IN THIS

THE ONE TRUE SECRET OF
LASTING WEIGHT LOSS

Karen Nimmo

RANDOM HOUSE
NEW ZEALAND

A RANDOM HOUSE BOOK published by Random House New Zealand
18 Poland Road, Glenfield, Auckland, New Zealand

For more information about our titles go to www.randomhouse.co.nz

A catalogue record for this book is available from the National Library of
New Zealand

Random House New Zealand is part of the Random House Group
New York London Sydney Auckland Delhi Johannesburg

First published 2009
© 2009 Karen Nimmo

The moral rights of the author have been asserted

ISBN 978 1 86979 175 9

Random House New Zealand uses non chlorine-bleached papers from
sustainably managed plantation forests.

Text design: Anna Seabrook
Cover design: Keely O'Shannessy
Cover image: Djordjo Grujica, BigStockPhoto
Printed in Australia by Griffin Press

CONTENTS

Author's note

While the letters and case notes in this book are based on the stories of real women, their names and identifying details have been changed or blurred beyond recognition. Where I suspected a woman's story might be recognisable I've blended details from several sources. Any attempts by my family and friends to see themselves in these pages are purely wishful thinking — except where I've pointed it out.

HERE'S HOW THIS BOOK CAME TO BE WRITTEN

I'm having a glass of wine with friends one evening when someone starts talking about weight. Okay, there's nothing too unusual in that. We are women. Obsessing about our weight is what we do. It's what we do even when we are out having fun. So my friend is telling us about this woman who's an acquaintance of someone she met at a work party.

'She put on 10kg after breaking up with this guy,' says my friend. 'He cheated with her best friend.'

'Bastard,' whispers someone else.

'And some best friend,' says another.

We all lean forward to hear the full story: possibly the one thing more interesting to us than our own weight troubles is the story of another's gain, especially when a man is involved. I know, I know, it's not an admirable trait but women will understand what I'm saying. Men shouldn't be reading this book.

So we're talking animatedly about this woman we don't know. Everyone has an opinion on her weight gain, as well as the guy (and skinny bitch) who caused it, what she should do to lose weight and what she shouldn't do. We cover which foods contain the most calories, whether carbs add weight faster than fats, whether swimming burns more kilojoules than walking, the merits of various fad diets. And so on. You know how it is. Don't tell me you haven't heard at least one of these conversations — if not, you really have to get out more. The reality is that modern women can tell you an awful lot about weight, diets, fat burning, exercise, kilojoules and all that goes with it. Not all of this information is correct, and virtually none of it has a scientific base, but that has never stopped us saying it out loud. Especially over a few drinks. But what strikes me, as I sit there, is that I'm not at all shocked by this conversation. You see, in an utterly weight-obsessed society, I've grown used to it. We all have. So have our daughters, and their friends. And it's absolutely crazy.

I've followed 'women and weight loss' ever since society, the media, and a whole lot of smart people known as diet and exercise gurus, started turning it into a mini-revolution. And I've been intrigued ever since I went on my first diet aged 18 only to discover that the more you focus on eating less food, the more you actually eat of it. Go figure. That set me off on a mission to find the ultimate answer to lasting weight loss, to find out why so few women successfully lose weight, why most of the others remain the same or seesaw up and down and even gain weight. And after all those hours of research, interviews and experimenting with programmes, you know what I found? ONE thing. Women who lose weight and maintain their new shape over time have just one thing in common. It's a secret that not only guarantees you will drop kilos permanently but also that you will lead a fuller, more meaningful life. And all you need to do to discover it is stay with me for the rest of the book.

Why is this programme better than all the others?

It's for women. Period. Many weight-loss programmes are developed by men. That's why they're based on problems and solutions: men like to 'fix' what's in front of them. That is, they take the problem (your excess weight) and come up with a solution (diet and exercise). They're less likely to consider why you are carrying the excess weight in the first place — nor what's going on in your mind and life that might be keeping it there. Don't get me wrong, many of these weight-loss programmes contain useful advice and sometimes they work. But ultimately they won't last for most women. If you are to get the most out of a weight-loss plan, you have to have one **designed for a woman**, and designed specifically for **YOU**. You have to have one that 'gets you': who you are, your history and your current circumstances. You have to have one developed to suit who you are and your life — not your weight problem.

This book has some new ideas. You don't have to buy any of them. That's okay with me; I'm not easily hurt by rejection. But I suspect if you are reading this book that other people's theories haven't worked for you so far — not for any length of time, anyway. So, on that basis, maybe it's worth a try? In summary, this is what this programme does better than others:

➜   Treats women as women — not as people or, more scarily, as men.

➜   Considers a woman's weight in the context of who she is and her life rather than as an isolated 'problem'.

➜   Targets the reasons a woman gains, carries and regains excess weight — instead of going after the weight itself.

➜   Lets you in on the one thing that has worked consistently for women who have lost weight and kept it off.

New research indicates that using psychology in weight loss leads to more long-term success. Among the psychological approaches now being used are adaptations of psychiatrist Aaron Beck's Cognitive Behavioural Therapy (CBT), which is used internationally in clinical psychology. It's based on changing the way you think and behave, to change the way you feel, in order to improve your life. This book uses a new combination of techniques taken from my research and experience in psychology, physical education and nutrition. While it draws selectively from CBT and other psychological models, I've developed many of the ideas and exercises specifically for weight loss and/or management after seeing what works for women — and what doesn't.

I want to say up front that using psychology in weight loss is not enough, you have to use practical physical strategies too because my goal is to have you **look better**, as well as **feel better.** Anything else would be a mean trick.

Be warned. This is not a diet book. It is not an exercise regime.

You won't have to starve, sweat buckets in a gym or wear anything made of lycra (unless that is your fashion fetish and if so you may need another kind of help). This book is about none of those boring things. It's about bigger, more important stuff. It's about figuring out who you are, why you carry excess weight, why your weight seems to be out of whack with what you eat and why, even when you drop a few kilos, they chase you mercilessly until you take them back. Most of all, this book is about change. If the word 'change' freaks you out, you should drop this book in the rubbish bin and head for the pantry. But if you believe change is possible, if you know you deserve to be fulfilled and you are prepared to do what it takes to achieve that, then it might be worth a read. So are you up for it? I thought so, or you wouldn't have gotten this far. Come on then. Make yourself comfy on my couch and let's have a little chat . . .

Why this book is not for men

This is what I love about men. Well, there are other things too, but this is a biggie. Men, in general, don't care about their size. Okay, I lie. Men do worry about the size of one of their body parts and they want it to be really, really big. In fact, if they could guarantee that food would bulk up that particular anatomical feature they would never stop eating. Truly, most men don't obsess about their weight. Only when they get to the point where they can't get past their stomach to find the TV remote control on the floor will a man note that he has a weight problem. Even then the panic will last about as long as it takes him to rip the tab off the next can of beer.

So you don't believe me? Try this test. Ask a man to name his favourite body part and I bet you he'll say breasts or legs. The enlightened man who realises you are asking about his body — not a female one — will look at you with a sly grin and a wink, and you'll know immediately what he is thinking. I mean, have you ever met a man who admits he takes size small underpants? Now, I'm not trying to depict men as Neanderthal beings who only drink lots of beer, wear bigger underpants than they need and dwell obsessively on sex. They do other things too. No, seriously, I'm just trying to point out the main gender difference when it comes to weight. Women obsess. Men barely care. They honestly believe that whatever their shortcomings they can pull the chicks. And, interestingly, they very often can. Men think women are gorgeous and are often surprised and confused when women don't see themselves the same way. And we are a lot more relaxed about the weight of the men in our lives than we are about our own. So guess who are the smart ones?

The point is that men and women think differently. I'm not talking about anatomical brain structure or hormonal differences, which may affect our moods and cognitive function. I'm talking about the content of our thoughts and the way we process them. More specifically, I'm talking about the way we view our bodies and weight and how we process societal pressure to be thin. That's why programmes that offer the ultimate answer to weight loss won't work for most women: they don't recognise men and women as different beings. It makes sense, doesn't it: women carry weight differently from men, mentally as well as physically, so we need different ways, different tricks, to lose it.

1 WHO NEEDS A BRILLIANT BUM?

'I've always wanted to be taller. I feel like a shrimp, but that's the way it goes. I'm five-foot four-and-a-half inches — that's actually average. Everything about me is average. Everything's normal, in the books. It's the things inside me that make me not average.'
Madonna

Here's the truth. You rock, whatever your size. You are special; you are unique; you are the only person who can contribute to the world what you can. Hopefully you agree with me. But your weight DOES matter. I wish I could write a book saying that any old weight is fine as long as you are happy with it. I can't though — I'd be lying. And although I have many flaws I'm not up for lying, not in print anyway. I don't need the hate mail.

Your weight matters because it has an impact on your health and physical appearance, and your physical self is a reflection of who you are — and how you think of yourself. However, what you weigh and how you look is not the most important thing about you. Not even close. Hold on, I hear the television presenters, actors, rock stars and models screaming: 'Our careers depend on the way we look.' Well, yes, that's true and that's why it takes a special woman to remain cool when people are rating her on her appearance (see why so many actors and models see therapists?). But here's the point I really want to make: our bodies are only a partial expression of all we are. If the essence of your being is your physical appearance, if your self-worth is based on your looks — and even your job — then you are in trouble. I don't care who you are, how much money you have, or how big your public profile. It comes down to a choice: you can focus everything on your body and be totally miserable (believe me, some of the most beautiful people in the world are the saddest). Or you can throw yourself into having a great life and make your 'look' part of that. There's no exchange voucher on your exterior so you might as well get used to it. Ultimately, you have two choices: you can turn yourself into a psychological wreck by hating your body or you can accept it and turn it into something you are proud of. There's nothing wrong with wanting and striving to look great — as long as it's not the focus of your life; as long as you have the other building blocks, the more important stuff, in place first.

Do you (really) need to lose weight?

Here's a true story. I know I said I wouldn't write about friends but I don't always stick to the rules. Even my own.

So I'm sitting in a café when the friend I've been waiting for walks in. No, that's wrong. She sweeps in. She's had her hair cut and coloured; she is wearing something dark and flattering; she has lost weight. Her eyes are sort of sparkly like she has just met a new man. I glance at my watch and think to myself that this could be a very long lunch but, of course, I don't say so. I'm a friend, remember. I concentrate on how terrific she looks and I tell her. I do it sincerely because she really does.

'I've lost a few kilos,' she says before spilling forth about the new man in her life (yep, there is one) and how well it's going. Then she says something that absolutely startles me.

'Just 10kg to go. If I could just lose 10kg more I'd be really happy.'

You've got to be kidding, I think. Here's this beautiful, talented, fun woman who always had men lapping at her feet, not to mention her other body parts, thinking a 10kg weight loss is her passport to happiness. And I say so, in the kindest way I can come up with.

'But you look great right now. Really great.'

'Yeah but . . .' she says then goes on to say how she's afraid that this guy will turn out like the last guy and the one before that.

And, well, I don't need to tell you that she had linked her experiences with these men to her weight. And, somehow, she had decided that 10kg was going to make all the difference this time. Of course it wasn't. Sadly, it didn't work out with this guy, possibly not because of the way he viewed her, but the way she viewed herself. The point is that my friend was fabulous just the way she was but, like most of us at various points in our lives, she just couldn't see it.

So the first thing to ask yourself is whether you actually need to lose weight. A lot of women don't — they just need to tone up what they have — and we'll get to that later. A lot of other women who could do with losing a little weight talk about it constantly but do absolutely nothing about it. I've done it. I bet you've done it. In fact, I can't think of many women who haven't. But, sadly, talking is often our preferred state. We like talking about our weight and — give us a break — talking is a whole lot easier than eating celery sticks and pumping iron. But I'm not about to lecture you on why you should stop talking about your weight and start doing something about it. That's what a man writing this book would do: give you a lecture on taking personal responsibility and taking action. Not me, though. I have many faults but being a man is not one of them. (Sorry guys. That was a joke. But what are you doing still reading this?) The thing is, we women know only too well what we should be doing with our mouths when it comes to weight — and it's not talking. It's not that easy though, is it?

The trick is to go back to the starting line and get a realistic handle on our weight. Do we need to lose weight and, if so, how much weight loss should we be aiming for? Or is it just a matter of toning up and getting rid of the stomach-clinging, thigh-pinching clothes that we think will make us look thinner when they are actually doing the polar opposite? Or ditching the baggy-shirts-over-leggings look that only worked on pregnant women in the 1990s? (Okay, maybe they never worked then either, but I don't want to hear that.)

In essence, there are **five** things to consider before you even begin to think about weight loss:

1.   Weigh in: where are you at right now?
2.   Rate your weight: how much is too much?
3.   Going up: what is your rate of gain?
4.   Why do you want to lose weight?
5.   What is the state of your life?

1. Weigh in: where are you at right now?

Mirror

Look at yourself. This sounds obvious — that's because it is. The first thing to do when assessing your body, weight and size is to look in the mirror. You can tell what's going on with your body just by looking at it, if you're honest. And when it comes to analysing our bodies, most women are far more than honest — we're brutal. Leave your clothes on when you do this because this is how most people see you, unless you have nudist beliefs or quite anti-social habits. The trick is to look at your **whole self**. Your hair, your face, your smile, your clothes, the whole lot. Women often don't realise that the 'package' is more important than each body part in isolation; they can't see their assets because they are so busy thinking about the 'problem' areas. We get all screwed up psychologically when we think our bum is a bit big when, in fact, it is in the right proportion for the rest of us. And if the same bum was wearing something a little more flattering, it could actually look good. Sometimes, of course, we really do need to lose weight but we need to be realistic about the extent of it. Before you step away from the mirror, think about how well your body functions. Is it strong and stable? Does it have plenty of energy? Is it supple and agile enough? Your body's ability to function at its best is a clue to how much, if any, weight you need to lose.

Scales

Now it's time to take your clothes off. Go to the bathroom or wherever you keep your scales, get naked, and weigh in. If you don't have scales and the nearest set is at the local mall, skip the naked bit. You don't need the criminal charges. But dress lightly and take off your shoes.

Check the time of day. First thing in the morning is cheating because you haven't eaten anything yet but that's fine if you have always cheated. At least you've been consistent. Okay, so you've got your weight. Write it down, along with the date and the time. Then I want you to take the scales out to the rubbish bin and drop them in it. If you can't do that, seal them up in a bag and give them to charity. Or give them to a friend, if she is not really a friend, and you want her to have the same struggles with weight that you have had. If you are sharing a flat then trashing the scales might lead to trouble. But at least see if the person who owns them will keep them in their own room. Of course if you weighed in at the mall, none of this applies. All you have to do is avoid that store for the rest of your natural life.

Why such extreme measures? Because scales bind us to our weight. They define us; they remind us; they trap us. They have the power to dictate whether it's going to be a 'good' day or a 'bad' day. They stop us going out for dinner. They make us yell at our partners and kids. They cause us guilt and shame. They get in the way of us having fun. They can ruin our lives. They give our pre-teen daughters the same body image hang-ups as we've got. Come on, what good things do they do? Can you name any?

How about this then? I have known women who refuse to give up the scales, the daily weigh-in, because they act like a security blanket. This is how Mel, 38, explained it to me: 'Weighing myself helps me to keep control of my eating, to stop the downward spiral. Or maybe I mean the outward spiral!'

In Mel's mind, the thought of getting on the scales every morning was the reason she was able to control her eating. I understand that. But it's not smart. She's in the grip of her weight and will be until she makes a major shift in her thinking and behaviour.

Tape measure

Now take a tape measure. Measure your chest, waist, hips, each thigh and each upper arm. Record them. Now put the tape away. No need to throw it out; it is just something about the scales that means if they are sitting in your house you will be drawn to stand on them far too often. Just put the tape back in the drawer and forget about it. Now have a look at those statistics. Think about them in relation to your weight and your height. Do you really need to make radical changes? Or is it really about a few annoying kilos or deposits of fat in odd places? Is it just a matter of wearing clothes that suit and fit you better? Or shifting the distribution of fatty deposit around a bit? Try to be honest because your answer will make a difference to your outcomes.

2. Rate your weight: how much is too much?

That's a question only you can answer. If you tip the scales at twice the weight of others of similar height and build, and you are truly happy with it, we're all happy. Well, sort of happy. Before you go skipping off into the sunset with a backpack full of chocolate bars, please check that you are not at serious risk of heart failure, diabetes or any of the other serious medical conditions associated with obesity. I'm only just getting to know you but I don't want you to die that way. I don't want you to live the way obese people are forced to live either. It's not fun — actually it's exhausting and frequently humiliating — and, worst of all, it's stopping you from reaching your full potential.

Seriously, though, if you are clinically obese, this book is not the first step for you. No book is. You need to see your GP for a full health check because we want you around for a bit yet. Your best contribution is still in front of you and obesity is the brick wall you have to get past in order to achieve it. Your excess weight or gain may be coming from an organic problem, such as glands or hormones, something that will render even your most dedicated efforts at weight control futile. So . . . please . . . pick up the phone and do it. Find an empathetic doctor who listens. Not one who pinches your fatty deposits with stainless steel tongs, shudders when you step on the scales and sends you away with a photocopied print-out for healthy living. You deserve better. And, as we all know, doctors make you pay for better.

For all the wailing about our obesity epidemic, most of us don't classify as obese. Not even close. We could just do with losing a few pounds and toning the rest up. Perhaps, more importantly, we could do with the psychological lift we would get from losing a few pounds and toning the rest up. Or not. Yes, that's right. Some of us don't need to lose anything at all. We could just do with less self-criticism, more confidence and an investment in a few more flattering clothes. We could just do with getting over our weight and getting on with our lives. It's not easy though, is it? Especially not when we have spent every day since our early teens (or before) stressing about our weight, and, often, allowed the scales to dictate whether the sun is going to come out for us today.

So where do we start? First, let's talk about the two main (official) means of measuring body weight: the body mass index (BMI) and waist circumference.

Body mass index (BMI)

If you've been on the weight loss trail for a while you'll know all about the BMI. For the record, it's probably the best known and internationally recognised measure of whether you are within the appropriate weight range for your height and gender. If you want it in more straightforward language, it measures your body fat. When used for children and teens, it is often referred to as BMI-for-age. The limitations of the BMI are also widely touted, and these are the main ones:

→   It may overestimate body fat in athletes and other people with a muscular build.
→   It may underestimate body fat in people who have lost muscle mass, such as older people, former athletes and people who have had long-term injuries.
→   It may not account for cultural and ethnic differences in body fat.
→   It may be misleading for use with adolescents because of the variation in maturity rates.

If you know all about it, if you have already worked out your personal BMI, you can skip this section. But for those who haven't, here's how it works: your body weight is divided by your height squared.

$$\text{Weight (kg)} \div \text{Height}^2 \text{ (m)} = \text{BMI}$$

If you are closer to a computer than a calculator, you can have your BMI calculated for you in seconds by one of the many websites you'll find by searching for body mass index. Just tap in your height and weight details and there you'll have it: a number that, potentially, can make or break your life. Then see where you fit on the table below.

BMI

Underweight	Below 18.5
Normal	18.5 – 24.9
Overweight	25.0 – 29.9
Obese	30.0 and above

If you are relatively light and lithe, it's all good fun. You can locate yourself on the pretzel end of the scale and wait quietly (hopefully not smugly) while all your friends do the calculation and pray they will meet the criteria for 'normal' weight. Argggghhhhh. Can I tell you how much I hate that? Of course I can, it's my book after all. But I really, really hate that. Who decides what it takes to be a 'normal' woman? And I mean that in every sense, not just when talking about size or weight. We are all normal. And it's sad, really. Surely we should be striving to be anything but normal. Isn't the whole point of living to be utterly and completely abnormal (as long as we don't steal, maim or kill things); to just be ourselves? We don't though, do we? We just want to be like everyone else. We spend a lifetime trying to fit in — to a whole lot more than size 10 jeans.

What you need to remember about the BMI is that it's a benchmark. Just a number. As I said earlier, it doesn't fully account for different builds or different bone masses, or cultural diversity. If you want to work yours out, fine. If you want to use it as a baseline to assess your progress over time, that's fine too. But using it to gauge whether you are normal or not, that's insane. Please don't do it. Instead, give yourself a hug and read on.

Waist circumference

The other main means of measuring body fat is waist circumference. It's a guideline for figuring out whether the amount of weight you are carrying around your midriff is upping your risk of developing (and potentially dying from) serious medical conditions. Pear-shaped women have an advantage with this one because they are slimmer around the waist proportionally than the bum and thighs. But, generally, I think waist circumference is a better indicator for women than the BMI; possibly for men, too, but remember they are not the subject of this book. The reason it is so relevant for women is that the stomach region is where weight gain is often most pronounced, especially as we get older. When we are younger we tend to carry excess on our bums and thighs but as we get older, have children, hit middle age or menopause, weight tends to settle around the midriff. While some change in body shape is to be expected, the amount of change, and fluctuation, around the stomach is a fairly reliable indicator of whether you need to be doing something about your weight, or whether your rate of gain is too rapid or too great.

So what's 'normal'?

As I said a moment ago, words like 'normal', along with 'perfect' and 'ideal', make me shudder. Just in case I didn't make it clear enough up above, let me say it again: I don't want you to be boring old 'normal'; I want you to be yourself. No one in the whole world can do it better. So please bear that in mind as you read this.

Experts have failed to agree on the benchmark for waist circumference. Some say around 76cm; that is, if your waist is more than 76cm then you should be doing something about it. Others say approximately 90cm is a better, more accurate, indicator. Pinpointing the number doesn't matter too much: there are a lot of perfectly healthy, fabulous-looking women with large waist sizes. The more important thing to consider is the rate and amount of change. Rapid gain (over say a year) is reason to be cautious, and to ask what's going on in the rest of your life. Not only does a marked increase around your stomach mean you are looking less fabulous than you are capable of looking, you are compromising your health. That scares me. So, go on, be honest about the trends in your weight gain. You don't have to write down your waist measurement but it is worth remembering, particularly in the context of your rate of weight gain, which is next on my list.

Among young women there is now an increasing trend to carry excess belly fat. This is probably the best expression of the change over time in our diet and activity levels, and in our lifestyles. Fast food, and faster, less active lifestyles, have contributed to an environment that presents challenges for those trying to maintain optimum health. It's a concern for young women because teenage weight problems are indicative of weight problems later on. I know, I know, it's futile trying to tell adolescents to make changes now that will improve their future. They're about as likely to listen to me on the subject of their weight as they are to rush to the nearest bank and draw up a retirement plan. And I don't want to go there. If you're a mother, that's your job. I have a hard enough time dealing with my own kids. But the truth is this: once your body settles into a pattern of how and where it carries excess weight, it becomes more difficult to change it over time. So young women reading this, please be warned. And if you're a mother, or in a position to influence young women's eating and activity habits, you owe it to them to do it. Hold back on the nagging, though. They'll only listen if they like you.

3. Going up: what is your rate of gain?

Read this section: it's important. The key thing to consider is your rate of gain over the past year, two years, five years. Disregard any temporary weight losses and look at your base gain rate per year. So if you weigh 75kg and have, for the past two or three years, gained 2kg a year then, unless you make changes, you will continue to expand at that rate. In five years you will be 10kg more than you are now and you will either have a wardrobe full of very tight clothes or, if you have faced your fear, clothes two sizes bigger. Or you will be at home developing agoraphobia because nothing fits, you are too proud to buy larger sizes and it's not sensible to leave the house naked. Especially in winter. Are you okay with that? If so, good for you, go help yourself to a biscuit because if you can live with it, the rest of us can. If you're not sure, it's worth thinking about the Law of Cumulatives, which applies to every area of your life. That is: **the more you do of what you are doing, the more you will have of what you've got.** So if your weight is on an upward trend and you do nothing about it, you have to accept that you will keep gaining weight — you will get better at it, if you like — and so you will start doing it faster.

And sadly, it isn't just the weight gain over time that will undo you — it is your failure to control it. You will damage your body image and your self-esteem. But here's the good news: if you do something to change the rate, the feeling of success will be worth it to you 10-fold. You will look good and feel better. Great, even. And it won't be about the weight you lost. It will be about your mastery of yourself and the feel-good factor when you look in the mirror. Trust me, it'll be worth it.

Is there a medical reason for your weight gain?

Some women have biological or medical problems that cause them to balloon and make that excess virtually impossible to shift. Biochemical imbalances and medical conditions such as polycystic ovary disease, insulin resistance and thyroid problems have all been linked with being overweight. But the percentage of women who can peg all their weight problems to such conditions is tiny. It's just that the truth is much harder to bear. In nearly all cases, excess weight is due to the intake (energy in kilojoules) exceeding the output (energy in kilojoules). In other words, putting more into your mouth each day than you are burning up during that same period. So if you want to lose weight the only way is to change the ratio between what goes in and what goes out.

4. Why do you want to lose weight?

Put yourself on the spot. Think hard about why you want to lose weight. Is it to attract a partner? Is it to look better in your clothes? Is it so you can wear a bikini this summer instead of some skimpy fabric straining to accommodate you? Is it so your body doesn't wobble like jelly every time you come to an abrupt stop? Is it for health reasons? Has your GP given you a warning? Whatever your reason, it's really just a smoke screen. All you really want is to feel better about yourself. To feel amazing. Then all the rest will follow.

Think about this. If your weight didn't change at all but your attitude to it — and yourself — did, you would change. You would act differently. You would think differently. You would be more confident. See how much difference your mind can make? The problem is that mind and body are inextricably linked, maybe even more so for women. Although my evidence is largely anecdotal, men seem better able than women to separate their thinking, particularly in relation to their bodies. So a man might say: 'I'm a bit out of shape physically but I'm still a pretty good catch.' A woman's thoughts might run like this: 'I'm fat and I'm ugly so I'll never find a partner.'

Now I'm not saying that the key to your own personal happiness is to make a quick change to the way you think about your body. I'm not that stupid, and you're not that much of a sucker. All I'm suggesting is that it wouldn't take much physical change to get you thinking better about yourself. That's why those 'make over your body' programmes work, at least in the short term. People like what they see and it gives them a psychological lift.

It's also why Britain's Trinny and Susannah, of *What Not to Wear* fame, and Gok Wan, from *How to Dress*, are such megastars. They don't even mention the word diet. They just go to work on the 'look' of the woman in front of them. (T&S do it a bit publicly for my taste . . . my body image isn't bad but it'll be another lifetime before I go on national TV in my underwear.) And wow, see the results! See what a physical makeover does for a woman's self-esteem — although I'd like to see how these women look (and feel) after they've done their own hair and been shopping all by themselves.

There is only one true reason to lose weight — and that is to **feel** better about yourself. It's not about the weight loss. It's about the sense of achievement. It's about the sense of change. It's about having some control over yourself. It's about how you **feel** because you have lost weight and because you **think** you look good/sexy/attractive. Celebrity stylists use clothes to empower women. It works because they tap into our feelings about ourselves. And our vanity. And our shopping gene.

STUFF TO DO: WHAT DO YOU THINK OF YOUR BODY?

Stop screaming now. It hurts my ears. Try to concentrate on all your good points because, believe me, you do have some. If you have absolutely no positive attributes then you are the first woman like that I've ever met. Men on the other hand . . . please guys, I'm joking. However, you would not be the first woman to **think** she has no redeeming features. Oh no. Not by a long shot. You'd be surprised how fragile and/or broken many women's self-esteem is. Or maybe you wouldn't.

Anyway, what good would a weight loss book be without making you do some self-analysis?

Name your own least favourite, or most disliked, body part. Write it down and write down the reason why. Do it in the space provided on this page if this book is yours — but if you intend to share this book with friends, do it on a scrap of paper. Why should other people know all your secrets?

Stop writing now! You only had to write down one. Why do women find this exercise in self-criticism so easy?

Now look at your answer . . .

Have you written bum, thighs or stomach? If so, it puts you among 95 per cent of women in the Western world. The only reason that bums aren't runaway stand-alone winners is simply because they're behind us. We can't see our bum in the mirror unless we turn around. So it has a bit of freedom to do whatever it wants. The thighs and the stomach aren't so lucky. But basically we don't like anything that has the potential to carry excess fat cells and, naturally, this changes over time. Think about how many older women complain about fatty upper arms?

Now write down your favourite body part . . .

If you hesitated, then relax, you remain in the great majority: many women simply refuse to answer, say they don't have a favourite, or make comments like this: 'That's hard. I've never thought about what I like. I've only thought about what I don't like.' Or, 'Are you just trying to depress me?'

When pressed, answers will most commonly range from eyes and skin to feet, smile, tan and hair. Women with perfect breasts will say breasts. Naturally. Here's the difference between us and the other inhabitants of Planet Earth: men won't dwell on their body parts with fatty deposits. (Remember I am speaking broadly here, I don't want to diminish male weight problems altogether.) Men will often look at you quite blankly when you ask them this question — they simply don't think about whether or not they like their bodies. They are just their bodies. If they do feel anguish, it is enviably brief. Occasionally they might say they don't like their toenails or legs or chest but they won't be undone by it. As for their favourite? Well, we've already covered that. Wouldn't they be sad if they knew we were more interested in the size of their hearts than that particular external organ. Wouldn't they be shocked?

Postscript to the exercise: if you need further proof, try this exercise on the women in your family, or your friends. See what I mean? Dislike of our physical selves is a sisterhood.

The purpose of this exercise is not to make you feel bad or worse — it's just to help you assess your body accurately. Before you can go to work and start making a few changes you need to be honest about where you are at. And you don't have to be honest with me. I'll probably never meet you (although it'd be nice, wouldn't it?) so you can lie to me and cheat and I won't think any less of you. But don't bother lying to yourself. That's stupid. You have to look at yourself all the time so unless your house is without mirrors and you never walk in front of shop windows there's no escape. You do look at yourself in shop windows, don't you? Or is it just me?

5. What is the state of your life?

Small book, very big question. But there's no point in pretending that what is going on in your life is not influencing your weight. Of course it is. I've seen it over and over again: often the clues to why a woman can't lose weight, or keep it off, are buried underneath that big beast of a thing also known as her life. The first thing I ask a woman who seriously wants to lose weight is to tell me about her life: her job, kids, relationships, finances, anything — because, invariably, that's where the answers to her particular weight issues lie. I'm not just talking about current lifestyle or relationships either. The past — events, situations and people — can still be having a huge influence over the way you think, behave, and look.

Most women, when they hear this, let out a huge sigh of relief. They know what's going on. They don't need a psychologist to tell them. They just want to talk. Because while they've been lectured for years about taking responsibility for what goes into their mouths and how much exercise they take — no one has taken the time to have a think about everything else going on in their lives. Not even them. The simple truth is that **a woman's weight is inextricably linked to the state of her life**. That's why you can't throw a diet and exercise regime at a woman and expect it to work. It won't. If it does, it'll be a short-term fix.

Don't believe me? A lot of the time stress, depression, anxiety and various traumas are responsible for a woman's weight gain and/or her inability to lose it. A lot of the time it has to do with events or people in her past that she is unconsciously holding on to. And give yourself a break: a lot of the time women in a fast-paced, contemporary world don't even have time to think. It comes down to pure logistics: when you have no time to think, all routines around food and activity go out the window. Or, at best, they are erratic. In this book we'll have a look at the past — past misery — because it really can keep you stuck in relation to your weight.

Happily, there are plenty of stories about women who have lost significant amounts of weight after addressing problems with past trauma, abuse, relationships and other issues. Genuine life satisfaction is the key to maintaining your weight, but don't beat yourself up. Happiness is pretty elusive: how many people do you know who have the perfect life? That's right, it didn't take you long to count them did it? Now have a think about their weight. I'm guessing, actually I'm guaranteeing, that you rate their bodies and/or weight as enviable. See the link?

STUFF TO DO: THE ULTIMATE BODY

Yes, another one already: getting you up and off the couch is all part of the deal. This one is huge fun in a group but you can do it alone.

Close your eyes and imagine yourself with the ultimate body. Go on — see yourself as a supermodel or actress if you like. Borrow the body parts of whoever you fancy. So maybe it's Cindy Crawford's boobs, J. Lo's bum, Sophie Dahl's curves, Keira Knightley's height? Dress the body however you want. Close-fitting jeans? A little black dress? Killer heels? A catwalk creation? Clothes are personal — just as we all have unique differences, we all have unique wants and tastes. But, whatever body you choose, you've got to imagine your own head on it. See yourself? Let the image sharpen up in your mind. See the colours. Feel the fit.

Now here's the fun bit. I want you to walk around the room as though you are that person. If you must keep your eyes closed, first make sure there's nothing in front of you because I'm not insured for your domestic injuries. But hold the picture firmly in your mind. Feel how you are walking, a little bit loose, a little bit sexy. You are smiling too, and not just because you feel like an absolute fool. If you are having trouble, here's a tip. Walk as though you are a little bit in love with yourself. Not totally love struck! That's dangerous. We've all seen those women — the ones who look like someone has shoved a carrot you-know-where — and we know who they are; the kind of women who couldn't kick back on the couch with a bag of crisps and a bottle of wine, the kind of women we don't want as our friends. That's not you. Just be yourself. Feels good, doesn't it? That's what you want: the confidence that goes with knowing you look great. To feel sexy and alive. See why it's not really about the weight?

Now I'll make you a promise. If you read this book all the way to the end, if you do the things I am suggesting you do, you will walk like that — with your eyes open. And it will make you a magnet for other people. It's like the Mona Lisa smile: everyone wonders what that smile was about. But, in addition to being able to paint a bit, Leonardo da Vinci was a smart guy. He knew women: that's why he was able to create an artwork that has intrigued us for centuries. When I see that legendary portrait I think to myself, 'Mona Lisa just dropped 6kg without dieting, without exercising, and she just fell a little bit in love with herself.'

So, are you up for it? As I said earlier, this plan is not about diet or strenuous exercise. It's about change. And commitment. And about making a few changes, committing to them, dealing with them and managing them when the going gets tough. And doesn't that feel better than making yet another hollow announcement: I'm going on another diet. I'm putting myself on a sensible eating plan for life. I'm balancing my energy intake and output. Blah. None of that horrible, dull stuff. We are women, we have to re-frame how we think and go about these things. And I reckon we can do it a whole lot better than we've done it before.

Food for thought

Have you noticed how many self-help books have a list of brilliant, searching take-home messages at the end of each section? I don't want you to miss out on that experience. You've paid for it. Unless, of course, you borrowed this book. In which case, you are smart as well as thrifty. So what have you learned from this chapter?

You are not a man. And, although I like men, that is a good thing.

You are fabulous right here, right now.

You need to be honest about your body. But you don't need to go on national TV in your underwear to do it.

You may need to lose weight. You may not.

Whoever invented scales was mean.

Go easy on yourself: your body reflects the (past, present and future) state of your life.

You don't need a psychologist to tell you all this. But it helps, doesn't it? (Well, doesn't it?)

2 MY BUM WOULD LOOK BRILLIANT IF . . . I COULD FIND THE RIGHT DIET

'Diets, like clothes, should be tailored to you.' *Joan Rivers, comedian*

Who are you? Who do you want to be? Those are the questions I always ask women when I first see them — no matter what the problem — because it's where you have to start. With the woman. And with her vision of herself. If you don't know who you are and what you want from your life, **no one** can help you get there. Not even someone with as much good intent as me. If you don't know and understand those things about yourself, you're stuck — in all aspects of your life. And you won't lose weight. Okay, you might lose weight (if you pay for very good help) but you won't keep it off. Sorry if this is hard to hear, but I feel obliged to speak the truth. I've seen too many women devote hideous amounts of time and money to the torture of weight loss only to see it all come undone because they haven't addressed the big questions first. (By the way, don't freak out if you can't answer those questions just yet. Almost no one can. By the end of this book things will be different.)

I see women in my psychology practice for lots of reasons: depression, stress, trauma, grief, anxiety, eating disorders, relationship and sexual problems, family and career issues, obsessions, addictions and a range of other difficulties. No one ever calls and books a session to address weight loss. No one rolls up to the first session, sits down, and starts straight in on her unhappiness with her body, weight or size. Repeat, no one. But, aside from those with eating disorders (who want to talk about anything but their weight), **all** women want to talk about their weight. So if they don't bring up the subject after a while, I open the door for them. Gently. (I'm in the business of making people feel good, remember.) So I say something really, really deep like this: Are you happy with yourself? And I make sure I have tissues handy because women really don't like themselves at all. Their weight is just a physical expression of the problem.

Once the subject of their weight is on the table, so to speak, women can't stop talking about it. They'll often confess they've had an obsession with food, dieting and their bodies that began in their early teens, sometimes in childhood. They'll spill it all: overeating, bingeing and purging, emotional eating, ballooning or yo-yo weight, the list is long. If they only knew how many women say the same thing, they wouldn't frame it as a confession or a 'guilty secret'. It's just the way it is for women — and it's why I started going beyond physical methods to use psychology in weight loss.

I'd better explain. I started out some 20 years ago with a physical education background, which meant I was young and all full of innovative weight-loss ideas about how to exercise and what/how/when to eat. So I designed plans for women that physically targeted the weight. You know, slash the food intake and bring on the gym workouts. And it worked — but only when the woman had a **really big reason** to lose weight (like an upcoming wedding or a new relationship or a major health issue). But then . . . oops. As soon as that reason went away, the weight began to creep back on. Sometimes it came back frighteningly fast. Often they ended up bigger than when they started. And suddenly my weight-loss strategies didn't look so good after all. I got away with it, of course, because these women believed that they regained weight because they didn't have enough willpower. But the truth had started to dawn on me . . . weight loss was not about going after the weight. It was not about what was going on with the body at all.

Time to test my new theory. Brimming with new confidence (and quite a few years later), I threw myself into studying the role of the mind in weight loss, thinking it would bring me to an 'ah-ha' moment that would make me scarily rich and famous. Guess what? Lasting weight loss wasn't about the mind either. It is just not possible to lose weight by giving your mind a workout, or a thought transplant, and ignoring your body. Nor was it simply a matter of combining mind and body techniques to come up with the ultimate weight-loss plan. Oh no. It was an even bigger deal. It was about the state of the woman's life, her past, her present and her future. Ah-ha!

The wonderful world of weight loss

Help! I'm desperate. I've tried everything, every diet, every weight-loss plan you can imagine. They work for a while, I lose a few kilos then the weight comes back on — with interest! Other people lose weight and keep it off. Is there such thing as a foolproof diet? Do diets ever work?
Sarah, serial dieter, 41

Dear Sarah,
Diets do work. Seriously. They work when the moon is in the second orbit of Venus and the stars line up over Saturn and the tide is on the second cusp of the fifty-third day of the new moon. Okay, you know I'm winding you up. Diets can and do work, my friend, although long-term success can be hard to achieve. Diets can be useful because they provide us with some structure, sensible advice and early encouragement. But controlling your food intake is only part of the solution. If you don't deal with issues and stressors in your life, and make some changes to your thinking and behaviour, you might as well hit the fridge.

Let's talk about diets because they are the foundation on which the multi-million dollar weight-loss industry has been built. They are also (sadly) part of what it means to be a woman. That's because we have all tried them, over and over and over . . . even though we're smart enough to know that the reason we keep trying them is that they didn't work the first time. Interestingly, very few diets are called diets anymore: they've been rebranded as 'programmes', 'lifestyle plans' and 'systems', and some of them offer sound and well-intentioned advice. Fad diets, however, do not. Fad diets lure us with promises of looking like a supermodel in a week and we take the bait because it sounds **easy** and **fast**. It's not smart because fad diets are gimmicky, usually unsustainable and occasionally dangerous. People who design fad diets want your money. Some of them really believe they are helping you, which is nice. Well, superficially nice. I still think they are full of it.

Diets, and the concept of dieting, often get bad press: boring, complex, anti-social, quick-fix and rip-off are just a few of the descriptions that spring to mind. But there are good and bad sides to restricting your food intake so it's only fair to consider both:

1 Good things about diets. Diets and detoxification plans can be very useful to kick-start your efforts to lose weight because reducing or changing what you eat is a good foundation for change. They can also offer some useful rules or structure for governing your eating and activity. And even the tiniest loss can foster some belief and be an incentive to keep going. Perhaps their biggest contribution, though, is a psychological one: they make you feel like you are 'doing something' about your weight, which makes you feel better about yourself.

2 Bad things about diets. Diets are about keeping your mouth shut — or monitoring everything that goes in it. They can also make you so hungry that even stale potato chips taste good. Diets address the reason you are carrying excess weight from the outside in, instead of working from the inside out. So they target the way you look instead of the way you are and the way you think. They also force you to spend every waking moment thinking about food. Certainly it's true that you can't put whatever you want in your mouth and expect to lose weight or maintain a healthy weight. But you have to have a Big Reason to take charge of what you eat. You have to like yourself enough to make those choices. And liking yourself starts on the inside.

Are some diets better than others?

Research indicates that no one diet is any better than any other in terms of results, although every weight loss 'guru' in the land would have me shackled for saying that. And they would have a point because they all have their own weight-loss success stories and they all truly believe in what they are doing. Even the wackiest diet can probably claim some success if you look hard enough. That's why there's a diet industry. Whenever the industry's 'experts' discover someone who has lost weight using their diet they make, well, a meal of it. Especially if the woman is attractive. There are big stories in the glossy magazines, interviews, before-photos, after-photos. But notice how there are hardly ever any I'm-still-thin-five-years-on photos? That's because they're hard to find and not because they're still skinny. Okay, that's a bit harsh. But there are very, very few lasting success stories. Most women are back to their pre-diet weight well before five years are up and, commonly, they are bigger than when they started out, which is so psychologically damaging. We'll talk more about that later. For now, the fairest thing to say is that **when a woman gets on to a weight-loss system that is right for her, at the right time of her life, it can work — and it can last.** The trick is to have all the other areas of your life working in the same direction.

Celebrity diets

The media makes me sick. It's full of weight-loss success stories using celebrities who have babies, then are back in their size 8 jeans before they've changed their first nappies. Then they hand out diet advice. It's not real and it's very depressing for the rest of us.
Distressed mother of four, aiming for size 14 jeans

Dear Distressed,
You're right except for one thing. Celebrities don't change their babies' nappies. They pay someone else to do it. And that's not the end of their problems. I know, it's a pain to read all these stories but the media is just tapping into our vulnerability: they know how desperate we are to find the 'answer'. The thing is, the answer does not lie in the lives of the rich and mega-famous. Sadly. It lies in the lives we create for ourselves. (Size 14 is a good aim; I bet you get there.)

Celebrity diets are the hot new thing. You will know this unless you have been living a totally cloistered life in recent years. Find me the magazine cover that does not feature a famous woman's exposed body looking very good or very bad and I will reward you heavily. Just not with chocolate.

Celebrity diets are stupid because who wants to be a celebrity? (Okay, we all do. Even celebrities want to look like celebrities because they really don't look like we think they look without major airbrushing.) Celebrity diets are stupid because they are designed for people who can afford help from personal trainers and chefs and hypnotists and psychologists. Most of us don't have those financial means (if you do have, please call me). If celebrities want freshly cooked wild salmon they just call their personal chef from their poolside lounger or text the chauffeur to swing by the deli, after he's picked up the chilled bottle of Krug. We lesser beings, however, would have to tramp for hours just to find a river to toss the fishing line into. And even then it would be futile for weight loss because of the number of chocolate bars we would eat along the way.

Let's not be too mean about celebrities because the women's magazines would be seriously dull without them. And gossip rocks. But they don't help us out too much when it comes to weight loss: they perpetuate the diet industry because their pay packets, their next jobs, depend on it. And how they suffer for their art: pruning their food intake to raw fruit, celery sticks and crackers, and living in fear of the paparazzi jumping out at them every time they leave the house in their track pants. I wouldn't want to live like that, would you? On the other hand, you have to say mega-money does have its compensations. It might not be able to buy happiness, but it can get you a personal chef and a country club membership. And, if weight loss is your goal, that's an awfully useful start.

STUFF TO DO: WHAT'S WORKED FOR YOU?

Actually this is not stuff to do, it's a memory test. Roll back through time and try to name all the diets, plans, cleansers, schemes, tips and tricks that you have tried to lose weight. Write them down. (Actually, you don't have to do that. I have a problem with writing down stuff because I'm lazy and I don't like writing on my books because I worry that one day I'll need to sell them to buy food.) But have a think about how successful (or not) these weight-loss endeavours were for you on a scale of 1–10.

1   10
it didn't work at all for me   it worked and I still look fabulous
                                                (in which case I am assuming you
                                                    bought this book for your sister
                                                            but got hooked)

Now, have a look at the list, if you've written one. And think through your list if you haven't. Don't dwell on the failures. That's not the aim of this exercise; focusing on where you've gone wrong isn't a good idea in any sphere of your life. In fact, if your efforts at weight loss were all failures then quickly screw up the piece of paper and trash it. But consider whether any of these programmes have worked well (or more or less well) for you over the years and, if so, keep it in mind. You may be able to use it to help you later on when we get some other things in place.

The truth about weight-loss programmes

No matter how many weight-loss programmes you've tried there are many, many more out there to tempt you. Just check out the titles at your library or bookstore — or surf the internet. The range is extraordinary.

I don't want to write an exposé of all the different options out there. It would take up the whole book and, even if you could sustain the boredom of reading it, we'd both end up back where we started: sad and confused and not having a clue how to achieve lasting weight loss. So here's a summary of the most common types of diets as I see them. I've left out specific names because I don't want to get personal or mean. And I don't need the lawsuits.

Eat-little-and-often diets. Diets that encourage you to eat little and often may have some merit but they don't usually work because people adjust the rules: eating little and often gradually becomes eating lots and very often. And the main problem I have with this is: Do you really need to walk around with snacks in your pocket so you can eat lots of food all day long?

Calorie- or point-counting diets. In theory it's a good idea to watch what and how much you eat. The trouble is that these diets make you think about food all day long; they teach you to think of food in terms of numbers. Which makes them stressful to calculate. Especially if, like me, you always hated maths. It's easier just to pour a glass of wine.

Weighing food or portion-control diets. Although I concede that most of us need to reduce our portions, this just keeps us focused on the numbers. A big piece of chicken should be allowed to be a big piece of chicken. That's how it would like to be remembered. Not that I've asked.

Special food/meal diets. Diets that require you to eat specially provided foods, such as energy shakes or vitamin drinks or mushed meals, can be an excellent kick-start but you need a very fine transition plan to ease you back to 'normal eating'. Eating this kind of food for any length of time is just plain anti-social. Unless you have an utterly magnetic personality, no one will ever want to eat with you. You won't be able to keep it up and still have a life. Where's the fun in that?

Food-matching diets. These are diets that get you to work out what goes with what because the enzymes in this food break down the enzymes in that, and so on. Only good if you have weird tastes in food combinations. Like broccoli and bananas. Or garlic and pears. Also only good if you have a degree in biochemical science and feel like spending hours wading through food-tech books. I'd rather read a magazine.

Support-group diets. These often have very smart weight-loss plans, resources and tips and the camaraderie is great. But diets that ask you to weigh yourself in front of others are in the business of humiliation. Your whole self-worth comes down to that single step you take on to the scales. A key advantage of these diets is that you get to spend time with other women with a common interest. In other words, it's fun. You're paying for this fun of course but it's a healthier option than spending a couple of hours in the pub.

One-on-one diets. These are a cool idea because you get special attention from your own personal weight-loss consultant. The trouble is that they talk to you about food and exercise and weight-loss goals. They don't talk to you about the really big stuff going on in your life. Like that you can't find a partner. Or you have a particularly selfish one. Your troublesome kids. Your stalled career (or lack of it). In other words, your **problems**. And if they do talk to you about that stuff they are not really listening, it is just a trick to make you hand over your cash.

Eat-lots-of-one-food-type diets. Yawn. These are just sooooooo boring. If you are up for a lifetime of lettuce or celery or eggs then maybe you have a chance with this kind of diet. But my guess is that you won't be able to stick to that unless you think it would be excellent to have a really, really dull life.

Protein diets. Diets that focus on protein, especially meats, are expensive, boring and heavy on your digestive system. If you think that daily platters full of bacon, steak and cheese will fast-track you to the kingdom of svelte then you need a reality check. And some darn fine cholesterol monitoring — unless you were blessed with arteries the size of the Channel tunnel. Obviously these won't work for vegetarians either.

Vegetarian diets. Suitable for vegetarians. Obviously. But not so good for those of us who like a sausage on the barbie.

Starvation diets. Diets that cause you to starve are stupid and dangerous (see books on eating disorders).

Low-carbohydrate diets. Favoured by models and the celebrity fraternity. Cutting back your carbohydrate intake can be a sensible approach but cutting carbs out altogether will make you tired and sick. In the case of models, this is often a swanky name for a starvation diet (see point above).

Eat-whatever-you-want-and-still-lose-weight diets. Diets that claim you can eat whatever you want when you want and still lose weight are even more stupid. Let's hope you can figure out why.

Think-thin diets. Diets that say it's all about the way you think make some good points, but if you think you can 'think' yourself to a 10kg weight loss then, well, it might be time to rejoin the rest of us on planet Earth.

Lose-weight-as-you-sleep diets. Diets that say you can lose weight in your sleep were invented by people who want to sell beds.

Country (insert name here) specific diets. Many countries have their own favourite and they might work if you live there. So, French diets are good if you live in France. Most of us don't want to spend that much time in our gardens looking for snails. Ditto Japanese diets. But we're talking about oceans and fish.

Medication diets. In other words, taking a pill to suppress your hunger. These are best described with five words. Chemical. Side effects. Expensive. Cheating. (Okay, the cheating doesn't matter but the other things do.) And what happens when you run out of pills? Or money?

A brilliant bum: the one true secret diet. This one works. But I would say that, wouldn't I? You're going to have to read right through to the end of the book to figure out how.

Food records

Yawn. Sigh. Food records or inventories are built into nearly all weight-loss programmes in one form or other. The idea is that you have to know exactly what you're putting into your body before you can do anything about changing it. Fair enough: any psychologist will confirm that having a really good grip on the problem is half the solution. There is a problem though . . .

Consider this. You go to a weight consultant. You are given a food record sheet to fill out over a week. It requires you to make an inventory of all the food you eat in any given day, then bring it back a week later and go through it, bit by bit, working out what is good, what is bad, what can stay, what has to go. It sounds all very scientific and workable but experience and research has taught me that it is also absolute bollocks. Why? Because it's boring and depressing to think about what you eat (especially when it is too much). **And because women lie.** We really do. Okay, some of our lies are well intentioned and some are wishful thinking, like we just 'forgot' about the bag of chips we sneaked when cleaning the pantry or the coffee (and cake) we squeezed in with a friend on Thursday or the bowl of ice cream we team with a night in front of television. Sometimes we actually do forget because we are so **bloody busy** doing everything for everyone else in our lives. So, food records, as an accurate record of what and how much we are eating, are practically useless. I've given up. And besides, it doesn't really matter what you did in the past — or are doing now — whatever it was, it hasn't worked. What you need to do is make some new rules. Dwelling on the past — especially a past with poor results — will bring no benefits. If you want benefits, you have to create a new now — and, therefore, a new future.

The key to making changes is to have an accurate baseline of **why** you are carrying excess weight, **why** you have gained weight or are continuing to gain and **why** you have struggled to lose it. In other words, it's not so much an inventory of what you are eating that you need, it's an inventory of who you are, what's happened in your life and what's going on right now.

These are the key reasons women are overweight, research and personal experience tells me. In brackets I've put the estimated proportion of women with weight problems who are affected or potentially affected;

→ Organic/health problems (hardly anyone).
→ Hormonal fluctuations (some, but potentially everyone).
→ Energy/food intake being greater than energy/activity output (everyone).
→ Life stages — post-pregnancy, middle age, menopause (many, but it's often an excuse too).
→ Misery (everyone).
→ Boredom (everyone).
→ Stress and lack of time/being too busy (everyone).
→ Low self-worth/esteem (everyone).
→ Lack of meaningful goals and viewing your future as boring (mind the avalanche).

Look at that list. It summarises why focusing solely on diet and exercise won't work. Notice how many things on that list are based on psychology or a woman's mind. What's great is that these are all things that can be changed. What's scary is that they can only be changed if you are ready. Ready to take charge — not of your weight, but of your life.

So are you ready? It's time to take responsibility for yourself. Our society encourages victims, to blame everyone but ourselves for boring work, no work, boring relationships, no relationships, our families, our finances, our lifestyle and — finally — our weight. When it comes to your body you have two choices: be a victim or not. Look in the mirror. Ask yourself honestly: 'Can I live with what I am now? Can I achieve happiness the way I am now?' If you answer yes to both questions, put down this book and go out for coffee. With cake. If no, then you'd better stick with me for a little while longer.

Here's my promise to you. If you follow a few simple rules that I will set down in later chapters, and make a few adjustments to the way you think (about food and activity, but mostly **yourself**) then you will succeed. You will look good and feel good. Wonderful, even. Wouldn't that be something?

Who are you? What do you love to do? What are you good at?

That is what I **want** to know. That is what you **have** to know. If you can't get excited about yourself and your future then what's the point of losing weight? Actually, let me answer that: there is no point. Who are you losing weight for? The only worthwhile answer to that is 'myself'.

Food for thought

Anyone can lose weight.

(Therefore) you can lose weight.

Many diets are stupid and unsustainable. We still try them, in the hope they will work.

Some diets can work. But only if you sort out your life at the same time.

Even celebrities want to look like celebrities.

Food records don't work because you will lie. Not because you are a bad person. Because you are busy and you are a woman.

If you don't know who you are and what you want, you won't lose weight permanently. So let's start there.

STUFF TO DO: THIS IS WHAT YOU ABSOLUTELY HAVE TO DO

Notice that this exercise starts on a new page. That's because it's really important and it deserves a page all of its own. Of course, like all of the Stuff to Do, I'll never know if you do it but, of all the demands I'm going to make of you in the pages ahead, this is the MOST IMPORTANT because this is the starting point of you looking as good as your genetic package allows.

You're going to set yourself a goal. It's not a weight goal in kilograms or a measurement in centimetres. We're not playing a numbers game; that's a guy thing and we need to do it differently this time.

Grab some old magazines and flick through for a body that you'd like to have. Find one that roughly echoes your own biology but is in better shape. Also look for a body that is wearing the kind of clothes you'd like to wear, then cut it out and stick it on a blank piece of paper. If you can't find the body and the clothes you like in one hit, cobble together your perfect form.

Then cut out a picture of your own head and stick it on top of the body.

That's you, that's your goal.

Now go and hang the visual somewhere you will see it often. Not on the fridge or in the pantry though because that's not where we want you spending the bulk of your time.

Why does this exercise work?

This is how **you** really want to look so it will slip into your subconscious and stay there.

This 'look' is realistic for you so you **will** be able to achieve it. When we aim to lose 10 or 15 or 20 kilos it's just a number to us, it doesn't personalise the goal. I am yet to meet a woman who sticks her head on a ridiculously thin body — because it just looks weird. And when skinny looks weird we suddenly don't want it as much as we thought we did.

3 MY BUM WOULD LOOK BRILLIANT IF ... I WAS LESS STRESSED

'Free your mind and your bottom will follow.' *Sarah Ferguson, Duchess of York*

Let's look at your life right **now** because it has such an impact on how you look and what you weigh. Not the past. Not the future. That's for later. First I have to get to know who you are, and what's going on in your life, right now. Some psychologists will start straight in on your relationship with your mother and how her issues (read: weirdness) had an impact on (read: screwed up) mini-you, but to me that spells trouble. Talking about your past before we fully understand your present is going to wreck your perspective. And whatever relationship you still have with your mother. The only reason to dig around in your past is to help you understand the person you are right now. Anything else is voyeurism and a little creepy. So let's not go there — yet.

Pretend that I'm your psychologist and you're coming to see me for a few sessions. It's a good deal for you. Even if you wouldn't pay real money to come and see me, I'm pretty good value for the price of a book. Even better if you borrowed it. It's not such a good deal for me because I don't get to meet you — and that's the fun part of helping people. Maybe, if I'm lucky, we will get to meet one day. In the meantime, though, we have to get to know each other through the only means we have available

— these pages — and I have to give you reason to trust me because that's the only way this will work.

I'm losing it! My life is crazy. I have no time to think straight. By the time I finish work I fly to the supermarket, grab the thing I can cook fastest, rush home, then cook and eat like I'm on speed — and that's on a good day. We end up having takeaways at least twice a week. I haven't been to the gym in months. I might as well have spent my gym membership on new clothes. Bigger ones. It's making me feel crazy and depressed. When will I ever get time to myself?
Stressed (and gaining weight fast), 34

Dear Stressed,
You're right. Lack of time is like swinging a wrecking ball at our best efforts to stay healthy. But having the perfect life that moves at the perfect pace is a myth. Who has one of those? Not me — and certainly not anyone who lives down here on planet Earth with the rest of us. But you do have time. In fact, it's all you have. It's just that you won't get any of it to yourself unless you take it. Sit down on a Sunday night and do some planning. If you can't find a couple of half hours for 'me time' in the whole week, I'm disappointed in you. Come on. You're a woman. Be devious.

The conspiracy theory

Yes, when it comes to our weight, there's a major conspiracy going on. In our minds, it's the world (the media, the environment, commercialism and modern life) against women. Everywhere we look, everywhere we are, everything we do, seems like a conspiracy to make us pile on weight — or feel terrible about whatever weight we're carrying.

Think about it. Society idealises skinny (and stigmatises fat) while encouraging overeating and quick-fix dieting. As the pace of life goes up, our physical activity goes down. Our environment is chock full of energy-dense (a euphemism for fat- and sugar-laden) food, which we eat in big portions and copious quantities because it's quick and available and we're in a hurry. Phrases like supersize, all-you-can-eat, to go and drive-through have become built into our language and our psyche. We eat big, bad and fast and our weight reflects it: one in three New Zealanders and Australians are overweight and the numbers are higher for indigenous peoples in both countries. While men are slightly more likely to be overweight, women are gaining more weight than men over time. For a long time, New Zealand and Australia have been able to hide in the shadow of the United States with its seemingly out-of-control overweight problems. But not any more, folks. We're up there alongside them. And the scary thing is that we haven't stopped growing. Not by a long shot.

Crisis time

Let me introduce you to my fabulous client. We'll call her Elisha. When I met Elisha she'd been looking after her unemployed partner who'd been off work for months with a head injury, she was working 60 hours a week to bankroll their debts and she'd recently had a late and devastating miscarriage. Her mood was low; she was tearful, irritable, constantly exhausted and figured she was 25kg overweight. When I asked her to write down her interests and what she was good at, which I do early on for many people, she burst into tears and bolted out the door.

I would have chased her but I don't run so fast in heels. I don't run so fast in anything, actually. So I called her instead and a week later she came back. And at the end of that first hour, after using my entire monthly quota of tissues, our conversation went something like this:

'I just don't see the point of all this,' she said.

'Living?'

'I don't think I really want to die but I've lost myself. Or maybe I never knew who I was.'

'Okay,' I said. 'How long do you think it would take to work it out?'

'Years,' she said, still weeping. 'For ever.'

It took four hours (over several weeks) — and that's not because I'm good; it's because she was. At our last session she bounded into my room in track pants and a muscle back singlet, her new energy barely contained and full of plans for her future. For the record, she didn't think she'd lost much weight at all. But she knew she was going to because she'd stopped worrying about it.

Elisha's story is typical of many women; the details of the stories are different but the way they present is very similar. They come to see a psychologist because they have hit their emotional breaking point, like Elisha did. But, usually, there are underlying problems with their self-image that can be tracked back to childhood or the self-critical teen years. The patterns that were set down all those years ago remain: I'm not just talking about food, eating and exercise, but also about the way women think about their body **and** about themselves. Over time, these patterns of behaviour and thinking become entrenched. And it's often not until a crisis occurs and they seek help that self-image problems reveal themselves. Of all the difficulties women present with, the one almost always lurking beneath the surface is poor self-esteem and associated low self-confidence. The good news is that it can be improved, sometimes rapidly. We'll talk more about self-esteem later though; first we need to consider what's going on in your life right now because stress has such an impact on us — not just on our weight, but managing our weight. That is, **what, when, how** and **why** we eat and exercise.

That crazy little thing called stress

Stress is good. No, really, it **is** good. It's just that in our crazy fast-paced lives, stress has had really bad press. Touted as something to **fear** and **avoid**, stress has become the monster of modern-day living. Lots and lots of people see psychologists, counsellors — and of course employment lawyers — for their stress-related problems. Even more people stay home, fretting, and don't get any help for them. When we are having a bad time of anything we tend to associate it with being under stress and being 'stressed out'. So the very concept floats on negative air: stress is depicted as a very bad thing.

So what is stress? Actually, do we really need to pull it apart? The structure of the word itself tells us everything we need to know: that it's a combination of strain and distress. It's also a modern term for acute anxiety. So far, so bad. But the truth is that stress is natural, normal, and it is integral to being fully alive. Think about it: many of the physical sensations associated with stress — racing or thumping heart, sweatiness, lying awake at night, butterflies in the stomach, struggles to concentrate, rapid and shallow breathing, whirling thoughts — are the same as those you feel when you're excited. Peak performance or function is dependent on feeling, and managing, some degree of stress: imagine an elite athlete trying to turn in a personal best at the Olympics without feeling some stress or pressure. It wouldn't happen.

Stress is behind women's greatest triumphs and achievements. Do you think Joan of Arc was in cruise mode when she led the French Army to victory during the Hundred Years' War? Do you think Marie Curie discovered radium without her fair share of frustration? Or Lady Godiva was all chilled out when she rode naked through the streets of Coventry to protest her husband's tax regime? Actually she probably was chilled out riding around naked in an English winter, but you get my point. Recall the last time you were excited (or in love) and how you felt physically: jittery and jumpy, keyed up, edgy, breathless, a little sick . . . see what I mean? The difference between stress and excitement is not so much physical as emotional and/or psychological.

Still, there's no getting away from it: modern lives are chaotic and some stress is toxic, messing with our psychological health, not to mention our best efforts at weight loss or control. Sometimes stress seems to be coming at us from every direction. Where is stress is biting you?

- → Work — no work, too much work or dissatisfying work.
- → Relationships — no partner or a partner you don't like or a partner who doesn't like you.
- → Social activities — too much on or a painfully empty diary.
- → Friends — tricky, self-absorbed or with endless issues, or too few friends.
- → Housework — everything to do with housework, if you are me.
- → Kids — where do we start?
- → Money — not enough (not too many people complain they have too much).
- → Health — sickness (like money, not too many people complain of excessive good health).
- → Time — no time to do anything well or poor use of time.
- → Weight — affected by all of the above (it's no wonder we have problems with it).

All of these stresses can occur without any sort of crisis going on. Any woman knows that it only takes one small glitch in the weekly plan to send the stress rating skyward.

How stressed are you?

Permanent weight loss depends on you having control of your life — not in a rigid way, but by being able to manage the bad days and enjoy the good ones. So you need to consider your stress levels and how you react to stress so you can work out how to counter it.

You've probably seen those checklists where you tick all the things that are going on in your life, then add up your personal stress score. You know how it goes: highest scores for family bereavement, divorce and/or separation, moving city, moving house, job loss and so on. The reason these are helpful is that they can explain and justify why you are feeling so terrible and that's a good thing. But these checklists don't account for the uniqueness of your situation, nor do they account for differences in the way we react to loss, disappointment and change.

How we deal with stressful events is entirely individual: some people shout and scream, some quake and shake, some keep it all locked up, some confront, some avoid. Don't be misled by those laid-back types either: even those who appear to barely break a sweat over anything may be stuffing their difficulties somewhere that may not be entirely healthy.

So how do we know we're stressed? I've listed below a few of the red flags. Remember that we all experience some of these signs or symptoms from time to time. But if you are experiencing clusters of these things — say five or more — you probably need to make changes. It's important to note, also, that feeling stressed can precede or indicate more serious psychological problems, which I'll talk about later in this chapter:

→ Changes in eating/exercise habits.
→ Body changes (weight increase, decrease or fluctuations).
→ Physical health problems (headaches, stomach problems, more colds, unexplained aches and pains).
→ Wakeful or disrupted sleep.
→ Feeling irritable and lacking tolerance.
→ Racing thoughts or going over and over a problem.

- → Struggles with daily routines, coping with work, domestic chores, study or kids.
- → Relationship problems.
- → Increased use of alcohol, drugs or cigarette smoking.
- → Extreme fatigue or exhaustion.
- → Excessive worrying in one or more areas of your life.
- → Feeling overwhelmed but lacking motivation.

STUFF TO DO: RATE YOUR STRESS

This is an easy one; you get to self-monitor and all you have to do is take a pen and draw a slash mark where you rate your own stress level — now and ideally. Just go on how you are feeling right now. Not as you lie on the sofa drinking wine and reading this book. But how you are feeling generally about your life.

What's your stress rating?

1		10
chilled out	medium	stressed out

What's your ideal stress rating?

1		10
chilled out	medium	stressed out

Interpreting the data (or what's the point of doing that?)
Nothing really, I'm playing with you. Seriously, though, this is just to help you see how you're feeling right now: under too much pressure or too little? My ideal is a fraction into the stressed-out side of medium, which is where I am on my best days. But this is not about me — and

we're all different. Some people thrive on intense pressure (although their cardiovascular system might have different ideas); some collapse under it. Your ratings are your business. But here's a basic guide that applies to both your current and ideal states:

8–10 = too wired and you need to reduce the stress levels right away. Even if you're a high achiever there's no way that under this amount of stress you can be having enough fun.

6–7 = so far, so good as long as you can stay in this zone. Most of us can't. A little pressure is generally helpful and can underpin peak performance, so don't be afraid of the occasional 8–10 feeling. Just make sure you get some downtime and avoid tipping into the high-stress zone too often.

3–5 = you're laid-back, which is a good thing. But take an honest look at your life. Are you excited? Or bored? If you are at peace with all that's going on in your life, fine. But when people read books like this it's not usually because they are fully satisfied. Maybe there's something missing. Perhaps it's time to figure out what it is?

0–2 = too bored and it's time to get off the sofa. And hurry up. Or you'll be old without doing all you're capable of. Or even anything at all. I'm not kidding about this either. Boredom is as bad for you as extreme tension. Boredom will make you eat as much as stress does. Maybe more. And it'll take you to the same unhappy place. Maybe faster.

Now think about this. This is the important bit. What is the one thing you could do right now to move your stress levels towards their ideal more often? Don't try to nail down something huge or life-changing because you won't do it. Make it small and easy to achieve, something that you can achieve within one week. For example, a five-minute daily walk; plan a catch-up with a friend with whom you can have a laugh (no cake though); listen to music once a day instead of once a week;

delegate one more chore to your partner or kids (ask nicely though, the aim is to get a yes); say no to a request you would usually say yes to and then feel stressed by having to do it.

Whatever you decide on, write it down in the space below if that's your thing. Or don't if you're like me. But do come up with something. And then put this book down and go DO whatever it is that you resolved to do. Then come back and tell me all about it. Well, tell me about it in your imagination. Talking to yourself in public might present you with another set of problems.

Welcome back. You didn't put the book down and go do the task did you? That's okay, I wouldn't have either; I would have kept right on reading if it suited me. You've paid for this book and you're reading it. That's all I can ask. Just promise me that later on, or tomorrow at the latest, you will do one thing to reduce or raise your stress levels. You'll be surprised at the sense of achievement it gives you — not so much because of the act itself, but because it will give you a sense that you are doing something for yourself. And, if you don't do anything, be warned: if you can't make one small change in this area, then you're going to strike trouble later on. So now we've established how you're feeling about your life generally, we need to get a little more specific about what's really going on.

STUFF TO DO: HOW DO YOU FEEL ABOUT YOUR LIFE?

(Yes, you've just done one but these are what makes the book work.)

Take this quiz.
I reckon you know how this works but I've been instructed to make it

clear. Using the table below, put a tick in the box that matters. Note that I've left one space blank. That's for you to add anything that is of special importance to you.

How do you feel about your...	Bad	Low	Okay	Good	Fantastic
Weight?					
Physical apearance?					
Intimate relationships?					
Kids/family?					
Friends?					
Work/career?					
Sense of humour?					
Leisure activities?					
Self-confidence?					
Future?					
Home environment?					
Money?					
Personal/spiritual growth?					

Scoring:

Relax: no adding up is necessary for this one. I never liked maths, remember. For a topic this important I'm not into calculations and those little summary boxes that say: if you scored xx points your life is really great/horrible. If you want that kind of quiz check out the internet or one of the glossy magazines. And if you want a much more serious take on the state of your life, there are many big, earnest books in the library or the book store that will help you out.

That's not for me though, and not for this book. I want to help you — not tear you into pieces to analyse you. All I want you to do with this quiz is look at your answers visually. So look at the table. What leaps out at you? Do you see a pattern? Is your stress all related to one thing — or one person? Are there certain areas of your life that need a makeover? Does all of it? Where is the biggest problem? That's the stuff that matters, not some number that I allocate you based on your answers, because that's where we need to make changes. You've probably heard it before, but I'll say it again because it's really, really important: the key to making changes in your life is to **do things differently.** If you expect radical new outcomes (or a new **you**) while continuing to do the things you've always done, then I can't help you. Sorry.

Note: You'll see that I've asked you to measure your sense of humour. If that seems a bit random, bear with me. When we're stressed or feeling down or exhausted, one of the first things to fly out the window is our sense of humour. It's one of the tests I use when assessing clients for the first time. I try to say something funny. (Give me a break, I said 'try'.) Most people get a joke. Even mine. People who are really stressed or depressed will barely notice, they'll just talk right through it. When people start chuckling in the sessions I know they're feeling better; when they start to laugh I know they're on their way back.

Serious stuff

I'm a clinical psychologist so a lot of the time I'm assessing people for serious mental health issues. So don't get sidetracked by the laughing thing. It's okay for psychologists to laugh and I like to do that very much. But just because I'm up for a joke doesn't mean that I'm not paying attention to the real — and sometimes serious — psychological problems that are going on for people. Depression, anxiety and body-image problems are endemic among women with low self-worth or loss of confidence buried underneath. Most women don't seek help until they face a crisis such as a relationship breakup or family difficulties, grief, illness, miscarriage or some other kind of adjustment problem. One of the greatest benefits of these crises is that a woman gets to spend some time on herself, with someone who is working only for her.

Even though stress has such an impact on our emotional and physical health, including our weight, it is not listed in the diagnostic manuals as a clinical problem. That's probably because stress on its own is hard to quantify; psychologists would say it is better described as a range of symptoms that can develop into depression and/or anxiety or other serious problems. But that doesn't mean stress-related symptoms aren't having a significant impact on your life and, in turn, your weight.

Below are the key symptoms of serious problems. Again, it's not about adding up any scores. But if you are experiencing clusters of these things, talk to your GP who should be able to refer you to expert help if you need it. While your weight or self-image may be playing a role in these problems, there may be other, deeper causes. If that's the case, go and see a professional.

Note: Before you commit yourself to seeing a mental health professional, check their credentials. Serious issues need expert help, not someone with good intentions who trained at a weekend workshop. If you do go to see someone, make sure:

→ You feel comfortable talking to them (most important).
→ They 'get' you and the world you inhabit.
→ They get a really good understanding of your problem before they start treating it.
→ They do more than dwell on the problem or patch it up — they help you move your life forward. Because talking about what's bothering you is only the start. You need a gentle hand to start moving in the right direction and you may need help to figure out what that direction is.

Symptoms of depression:
→ Low, sad (tearfulness), depressed mood.
→ Sleeping and/or eating difficulties (changes in patterns including appetite or weight).
→ Finding it hard to do things — daily tasks and chores, work, study, look after kids.
→ Concentration and decision-making problems.
→ Constant or frequent fatigue/exhaustion, low energy, low motivation.
→ Getting no or little pleasure from usually enjoyed activities.
→ Decreased sexual interest/drive.
→ Feeling guilty.
→ Feeling worthless; self-critical thoughts.
→ Hopeless view of the future.
→ Withdrawing from people and activities.
→ Suicidal thoughts or planning.

Symptoms of anxiety:

→ Shortness of breath, rapid and shallow breathing.
→ Rapid heart rate.
→ Feeling nervous, panicky, restless and keyed up.
→ Increased irritability.
→ Stomach problems, constant 'butterflies', nausea, diarrhoea.
→ Trembling, twitching, shakiness, sweating (feeling hot and cold).
→ Avoiding places where you might be anxious.
→ Concentration problems.
→ Easily startled.
→ Sleep problems (can't go to sleep, night waking).
→ Belief that you are helpless/unable to cope.
→ Thinking something terrible/disastrous/life-threatening will happen.

Depression and anxiety can be quite hard to separate. Quite often, women demonstrate symptoms from both categories, which makes sense, doesn't it? If you are depressed you will probably be worked up about it and various things in your life. And if you are feeling uptight and anxious it's almost certainly going to affect your mood — in a negative way. What you are experiencing doesn't have to fit neatly into one box. If you are struggling to do things you would normally find easy or pleasurable then you should at least start to ask the right people about what's going on.

Problem eating and body image difficulties

Problem eating and body image issues can be hard to quantify as a 'problem' because so many women struggle with these to a greater or lesser extent. Yo-yo dieting or erratic eating, for example, counts as problem eating and women who love their bodies are about as rare as fat-free French fries. So it can be tough to figure out when these problems cross the line into serious territory.

I'm not going to talk about underweight conditions like anorexia nervosa here because these need specialist attention. However, we need to touch on other clinical conditions such as bulimia nervosa and binge eating because they can be present in women who perceive themselves as overweight. Again, these are complex issues but it's worth noting the key signs and distinctions. Some of the reasons these problems develop are discussed in later chapters.

Bulimia nervosa and binge eating

Officially, bulimia nervosa affects one to three per cent of the population although many more women suffer to various degrees. It usually begins in adolescence or early adulthood, often after a period of dieting. Bulimic women tend to be of average weight, or slightly overweight, yet extremely distressed by their weight. Depression is often present in these women.

Bulimia is characterised by binge eating and the use of strategies to 'undo the damage' such as purging/vomiting, fasting or excessive exercise. To be classed as a disorder, this must occur at least twice a week for three months and, invariably, the woman's beliefs about her body weight and shape fuel negative self-beliefs. Bulimia can persist over many years or have a stop-start pattern. While body dissatisfaction doesn't seem to increase with age, it often doesn't go away either. Not surprisingly, we're starting to see an increase in women with midlife eating disorders because women who are now 40–55 years old were the first generation to be seduced by the 'culture of thinness'.

A 'binge' is consuming more food than most others would in the same period — usually it's less than two hours. The food is most often sweet or high-calorie although bingeing is more about the amount of food than a craving for a particular type of food. Binge eating is usually done in secrecy, may feel frenzied and out of control, and the person may eat until they are painfully full. Binges are most commonly triggered by mood states, especially feeling down, stressful events, intense hunger (e.g. after being on a diet) or feelings related to body weight and food.

As noted above, three strategies are most commonly used to counter bingeing:

→ Purging/vomiting — it is estimated that this is used by 80–90 per cent of those who binge.
→ Fasting — for one or more days.
→ Excessive exercise — classed as excessive when it interferes with important activities or is done at inappropriate times or in inappropriate settings.

It's important to note that while many women don't quite meet the criteria for an eating disorder, they may still be struggling and need help. Generally, the key to figuring out when your weight problems are seriously serious is how much they are affecting your life and ability to function normally.

To do that, ask yourself these three questions:

1 Does my weight/physical appearance — and constant thinking about it — stop me from working, going out and engaging in normal activities?

2 Does my weight-checking behaviour — weighing, measuring, mirror checking — interfere with me carrying out daily activities?

3 Does my weight (and thoughts about it) make me do things that compromise my physical health — starve, binge, purge/vomit, eat very erratically, exercise manically, take no exercise at all?

If your weight issues have made you unable to function, or put your health at risk in any way, then you should seek expert help. If you know someone who is experiencing these things, then helping them to get a professional opinion is the kindest and most responsible thing. However, if you are like the majority of women who experience degrees of these problems and reactions, then you can do an awful lot to help yourself.

Dealing with stress

Your stress levels negatively affect your weight. So you have to find a way to reduce or at least manage them or your efforts to lose weight will be beaten into submission by all the crazy stuff going on in your life. There are a lot of ways to deal with stress — and a lot of literature available to help you. I could fill up this whole book with strategic advice about stress management but I wouldn't be doing it better than anyone else. In fact, I'd probably do it worse because I'd get sick of it. So I'll just summarise the best ideas that everyone has come up with so far and leave the choice to you.

Breathing. Let's hope we're all agreed on the merits of breathing. That is, the only advantage in not breathing is permanent release from weight issues. With regard to stress, I'm talking about the importance of breathing through your abdomen rather than your chest. Most of us breathe too shallowly and this contributes to us feeling wound up and stressed.

Try this: sit in a chair with your hands on your stomach and take several deep breaths. Watch your hands. Do they rise with each breath in — or does your chest? If your chest is rising more than your hands you need to work on your breathing. It's worth it because it's a quick and effective way to calm yourself when you are feeling uptight.

Yoga, Meditation, Pilates and other breath control activities. I've never been a big fan of yoga but only because I can barely touch my knees from a standing start and I don't want to be found out. But the positive experiences of so many women are more important than mine. Meditation, in its various forms, also has many followers as does Pilates, which assists strength and flexibility. By using the mind to control the muscles, it seeks to promote your body's strengths, improve weaknesses and correct imbalances. The other idea is that proper breathing enhances blood flow to reduce tension and promote full body function. Full exhalation is touted as the key to full inhalation, which is a little different from the traditional approach.

Try this: breathe in deeply and then breathe out as hard as you can — until it feels like the air has been wrung out of your lungs. You should be able to note the use of your deep abdominal and pelvic floor muscles. If, like me, you don't notice any of that because you have started to cough then you have some work to do.

Relaxation. Progressive muscle relaxation is where you lie down and go through each of the muscle groups, tightening and then relaxing. Or visualisation where you see yourself on a beach or a park and the associated good feelings flood your body. These techniques work and, again, hundreds of thousands of women could vouch for them. But I don't find it all that practical to lie down in the middle of a shopping mall or on a busy street to ease my stress.

Note: New research has touted relaxation techniques as a solution to weight problems. These can help but we need to make a careful distinction here. Dealing with the stress in your life will help you lose weight. Lying around clenching your muscles and thinking about beaches will not.

'Me' time. Includes a hot bath, good magazine, time with the iPod or a book. These are great if you can get past the stress of thinking that you're just wasting time.

Sex. This may well be the greatest antidote of them all. Depending on who's available to do it with. So look around you. If there's no one exceptional within reach, you might like to file this one under 'me' time — if you get what I mean and I'm sure you do.

Friends. To my mind, this can be better than any of the above. Even sex. Anyone who has been on a raucous girls' night out or girls' weekend will confirm this. If you haven't, it's a good thing to aim for because time spent laughing with friends can be utterly rejuvenating. But be a little choosy about the company. Some people exude potential for good times but in reality they're just exhausting because they have so many **issues**. Let them be someone else's friends — not yours.

Fun. This is a daily necessity. If you're not having any fun then something about your life needs changing. Seriously. Isn't having fun the whole point of everything?

Food for thought

Some stress is good. Some stress is bad, even toxic.

Toxic stress can affect our psychological health. And our weight.

Toxic stress can lead to serious psychological issues. Seek help if you need it.

Being busy isn't a reason to be overweight. But it's a good excuse.

Relaxation helps but you won't lose weight lying on a beach. You may even gain it.

Time is all you have. Do good stuff with it.

Fun is the best antidote to stress. Are you having any?

4 MY BUM WOULD LOOK BRILLIANT IF . . . I HAD SKINNY GENES

'I don't think I could be a wallflower with a body like this.'
Sophie Dahl, curvaceous model

Here's what happens: you start life with a biological blueprint for your physical self. You are fine with that for a few years. Toddlers don't have body image issues, thankfully. Time passes, sometimes happily, sometimes not. Then you grow up, and out, and find you don't much like the look of the person staring back at you in the mirror. Oh no, you think, cursing your blobby genetics, your snail-like metabolism, your family's love of deep-fried food. **My body is their body. They set me up for this. It's all their fault.** And, in your subconscious mind, two things begin to happen without you even noticing:

1 **You accept it.** As you slowly gain weight, you start to feel your adult size is inevitable. You start to see yourself as a big person, perhaps just like everyone else in your family, perhaps because someone once told you that you have 'big bones' or called you 'fat'. You begin to think and act as if you are already that size. And guess what happens to your weight? That's right. It slowly increases to the level your mind has already set for it.

2 **You fight it.** Just because you subconsciously accept
something as inevitable, doesn't mean you like it. You
desperately resist gaining weight. You start to think about
everything you eat (and don't eat). You cut back your food intake.
You may exercise frantically, then stop. Or you do nothing at all.
You feel guilt, fear and panic. Every waking moment (well, way
too many of them) begins to be spent in the fight against gaining
weight. And the more you focus on not gaining weight, the more
you put on.

The clash of these two thoughts sets up an internal conflict around food
and losing weight from which you get no respite. I should not, I must
not . . . versus, I might as well, I'm going to put on weight anyway.

Welcome to the nightmare.

Blaming the family?

Biological factors, such as your genes and your metabolism, play a
definite role in making up your physical being. There's no hiding from
that. But it's time to stop yelling at your mother. That's the coward's way
out. It's always easier to blame someone else for your problems than to
take responsibility for yourself. And it's much, much easier to blame
your mother for your weight than to leave the cake on the plate or go out
for a brisk walk in the rain. Besides, mothers are safe targets because
when it comes to our kids we are full of guilt (if you're not a mother
already, then just you wait).

In overweight people, height, bone size, body mass, fat-storage
capacity and metabolism all have a hereditary component. Studies
indicate that having overweight parents hikes up your chances of being
overweight yourself — about 25 per cent increased odds if one parent is
overweight, and up to 50 per cent if both are. But remember — it's not
just your parents' genes contributing to those statistics or the way you
look. It's also got a whole lot to do with the food/activity environment
that you were raised in. The habits and thinking you form around food
and activity as a child often stay with you. So the kinds of foods you ate,
when and how often, the size of portions, your fast food/sweets intake,

how active (or inactive) you were, how active you were encouraged to be, have all contributed to the way you look now.

But you know what?

A far bigger contributor than all of those things to the way you look now is **the way you think now** and the **things you do now.** And these are things you can change — if you choose to.

What about culture?

Different cultures are associated with different body shapes and sizes. No surprises there. But it's not so important to recognise that there are cultural differences as it is to understand that there are many reasons for them. Genetic make-up is part of it; so is a culture's perception of appropriate body size (some cultures favour large women over thin), diet and the way food is used in rituals, ceremonies and celebrations.

In Australia and New Zealand, cultural differences in weight norms and expectations, eating patterns and behaviours are evident. Indigenous peoples — Maori and Australian Aborigines — are more likely to be overweight than the broader population. Pacific Islanders living in New Zealand or Australia demonstrate more weight problems than those living in their home countries because their diet tends to be traditional cooked food supplemented with the best (or should I say the worst) from the West.

Women from these cultures, who are on average a few kilograms heavier than their sisters of European descent, face some specific difficulties with losing weight. These need to be looked at as challenges though — not reasons to give up:

> **Celebrations.** In some traditional cultures, many get-togethers are organised around feasting. Providing/bringing food is a way of showing respect and hospitality to others. To not partake would be ill-mannered and frowned upon. Which is all very well, but it makes it difficult for a woman who is trying to control her weight. Let's face it, it's much easier to eat and be loved than the other option. So guess which one we're always going to take?

Cooking style. While Europeans generally cook enough food for the family meal, that's not necessarily the approach for other ethnicities. For example, Maori and Pacific Islanders tend to cook so there are leftovers for later on, the next day or if friends and relatives turn up unannounced (which they regularly do). So it's hard to deny yourself when there is plenty of tasty food available all the time.

Weight norms. In ethnic groups where it's seen as more socially acceptable and often attractive for women to be large, they are likely to be large. And if the people you spend the most time with are bigger, you are more likely to be bigger. Your choice of clothing makes a difference too: it's easier to 'grow' if you are always in relaxed, flowing clothes.

Food type. Traditional Pacific Island food is hot, cooked, starchy and often flavoured with coconut cream. Salads have never been important traditionally, and green vegetables are less commonly used than in European society. So the diet is not compatible with weight loss or maintenance, especially not when topped up with a late night visit to KFC.

I'm worried! My grandmother was big. My mother and her sisters are big. I'm getting bigger. I'm Samoan and my family is full of overweight people: men and women. Every family occasion we have is built around food. I've tried heaps of diets but none have worked for any serious amount of time. Trying to lose weight feels futile. A big, fat waste of time. I'm going to end up looking like my mother and my aunties anyway. Should I just give up and be happy with myself as I am?
Sina, 38

Dear Sina,
You know what? I'd say give up the fight in a heartbeat if I thought it'd make you happy. It won't though, will it? I don't know you but I'd say your weight stresses you out every day of your life, which

*therefore puts you among 98 per cent of the female population.
I get that it's hard for Pacific Island women living in New Zealand
or Australia because you have to walk the line between the two
cultures. Sometimes, there's taro for lunch and there's KFC for
dinner. But you don't have to be like your mother or your aunties
— or eat like them. You can choose. If you want to, you can do
things differently. But it's over to you. I can live with your weight if
you can.*

Other cultures

I've touched on Polynesian cultures here because weight problems are so prevalent among these women — and they're increasing at an even faster rate than among women of European descent. A full exploration of cultural weight difficulties is beyond the scope of this book, but I acknowledge women from a raft of ethnic backgrounds are fighting the same battles. These battles are tougher for women living in the West who have to manage the clash between their own food and lifestyle traditions and those of their adopted countries. And when they take up the excesses of each, their bodies are really in trouble.

You and the fruit thing

On the subject of culture, you've heard this before. Me too, and I'm kind of sick of it. Australian and New Zealand women of European descent are traditionally said to be pear-shaped: that is, we have bigger bums and thighs in relation to our chests. It's an evolutionary thing that apparently goes way back to our pioneering past, although I've never figured out exactly why we needed all that lower level bulk at the expense of breasts. Maybe big breasts would have messed up our butter churning? Who knows? What we do know is that there's been an evolutionary update: now we're told that as our national average weight increases Antipodean women are turning into apples. (Who comes up with these fruit analogies for women's bodies? It must be a man trying to be kind. Without success.) Anyway, being apple-shaped means you're round between the neck and the knees, which doesn't seem to me like a good reason to throw a party.

Apple-shaped bodies are very American — and Americans tout

themselves as the biggest and the best of everything. And when it comes to bums their opinions carry a bit of weight. Apologies to any Americans reading this but you guys are real big and super-size everything and we want to pretend that we're not and we don't for a little longer. Even in denial, though, we probably have to concede something to the apple thing: that the size of our chests and especially our stomachs on the increase to match the rest of us. And the age at which we start noticing it is going down. Way down to the early teens, and sometimes even earlier.

Your past

In order to understand you, we have to turn back the clock. We have to go way back to who you were (and who you were with) when you arrived on the planet. This is not voyeurism on my part, I swear. Some psychologists do that: work extensively with the child-like you. I don't. I only want to know enough about your past to understand your present because that's all I need to know. If I don't get pretty quickly to what's going on for you right now, we're in trouble. There's no point helping the child-like you to lose weight because she's all grown up now and she has a different set of problems. I want to help the woman sitting in front of me — or the woman reading this book.

But we do have to go back in time a little bit because our genetics, our parents and our history explains who we are. Women's stories are very personal. I've never heard two stories the same, but frequently the key to why a woman carries excess weight is buried in her past. Sometimes it can be found in her home or family situation, sometimes in her broader environment. The trick is to locate it. Because once you understand how your current beliefs about food and weight (and especially yourself) were formed, you can go about changing them.

STUFF TO DO: **YOUR PAST AND YOUR WEIGHT**

Here are a few questions to get you thinking about your past and how it might have influenced your 'relationship with food'. (It's a dodgy description I know, but I really can't think of a better one.) You can write down the answers if you want to but that's not the important thing. The idea is not to blame anyone, but to help you see the things in your past that might have set you up for a struggle with your weight:

→ What did your family eat? How? When? How much? How often? What were the 'rules' about eating and food?

→ Did you sit down to eat as a family, eat in front of TV or eat on the run?

→ How often did your family have takeaways? Junk food?

→ How did your mother think and behave in relation to food?

→ What about your sisters or aunties?

→ Did you eat the same way as your family or have different habits and patterns?

→ When did you start thinking of yourself as overweight? What led to or caused this?

→ Did you ever binge or eat secretly?

→ Did you eat when you were sad, stressed, bored or angry, or as a reward or punishment?

→ Do you still eat for any of these reasons? When? How often?

What do the answers mean?

Good question, but it can't be answered generically. The answers mean different things to different women. It's just a way of helping you understand yourself in relation to food, so look through your answers and see what jumps out at you. Are there any patterns? There are a few things to note though:

1 **Family legacies.** If your habits now are those of the family you were raised in — and they are not good ones — then you are comparatively lucky. All you have to do is change them, and change is possible. So keep reading.

2 **Emotional or comfort eating.** If that's you, a stress or sadness or boredom eater, then you need to change your life. You should keep reading too because there's a whole section on emotional eating later on (see chapter 7).

3 **The first woman in your life.** This is the bit where you're allowed to blame your mother or your primary female caregiver. Only a little bit, though. And no yelling. Especially if you're a mother already because, despite your best efforts to spare your daughters, you are passing on your own demons. Research tells us that women are particularly influenced by their own mother's relationship with food. So if your mother was a serial dieter, secret eater, bulimic or worried incessantly about her body/looks then, in ways you may not even notice, you will be carrying that legacy. Don't get too uptight about it, though, because women who don't have any food issues at all are a rare breed indeed. Note: If your mother was a woman with no food or eating issues, you are very, very lucky. You also have no excuse.

Now just some points on environmental conditioning because it's so important. When a girl follows her mother, female caregiver or female family members into a lifetime of food consciousness and dieting, it may well be less about genetics and more about the environment she was raised in. It can work in a number of ways:

→ The girl sees her mother as big or as continually fighting her weight. She thinks this is the size she is destined to be — and the battle she is destined to fight.

→ The food at home is plentiful because the mother likes to eat (maybe Dad and the other kids do too). They eat the same things and the same large portions.

- → The girl becomes food conscious in the same way as her mother.
- → The girl eats or restricts food or binges on food in the same way as her mother.
- → The girl adopts activity habits that mirror her mother.
- → The girl interprets media and societal messages in the same way as her mother did and does.
- → The mother repeatedly talks about the war against weight. The girl absorbs it. She puts on her shield and armour and prepares for the long fight against her body and her urges. And so the cycle continues . . .

So go easy on yourself. From a very young age you may have been conditioned to enter the minefield of food, dieting and weight. We can't help it: as women we put much of the pressure on ourselves. Media messages suggest to us that our dieting, the way we dress, is aimed at looking attractive to men. When let's face it most men would prefer you wore nothing at all and would be hard-pressed to tell the difference between current fashion and that of 20 years ago. Short, low-cut and tight works pretty well for most of them. So, in fact, with our bodies and what we wear, we are mostly looking to please other women. Which is seriously boring. Why not concentrate on pleasing yourself? And even if you are hunkering down to fight a war with food for the rest of your life, give your daughter a break. You owe it to her. Don't make her ride the rollercoaster with you. She will get enough pressure from society, the media, her mates and everyone around her to look 'perfect' without adopting your obsessions. Don't set her up. Start conditioning her to think that food is no big deal. If you need it, eat it. Unless it is her absolute passion, and she wants to be a chef, then food should take its proper place in the scheme of things. You need it to live, it can be enjoyed with friends and it's sometimes fun to cook — but that's it. It should not rule your day. I've had friends who refused to go out for dinner because it would mess up the diet that they were messing up daily anyway. Or it would mess up the diet they knew they should be on but hadn't quite started yet. Is that any kind of way to live?

Once you've finished with your mother, have a think about your expectations for your weight. If your mother had food and weight problems did you expect to wind up with some too? When you hit your teens and put on a bit of weight did you say: 'Oh no, it's my inheritance; here it comes, I can't do a darn thing about it.' It's fascinating, because many women just hand over control of their body — and ultimately their lives — to the food in the pantry, to the food in the fridge, to anything or anyone but themselves. It's like they were driving along in their car and someone just came along and said, 'Move over . . . I wanna drive your car and I wanna drive it for the rest of your life. I don't care if it's yours, move over.' What surprises me, absolutely fascinates me, is that women roll over. Quickly. They just slide across into the passenger seat without a backward glance at the keys, strap on the seat belt and say to the fridge and the pantry, 'Okay you drive. You drive my car for the rest of my life.'

If not the folks, then the metabolism — surely?

Metabolism gets really bad press, which is tough considering most people don't really know what it is. In simplistic terms, metabolism refers to the physical and chemical processes that break down food and oxygen to transform it into energy. Ah, food breakdown. No wonder it takes so much of the blame for women's weight gain and diet failure: if the food you eat is converting into body fat instead of energy it must be that freaking metabolism. There's even a name for it now — Slow Metabolism Syndrome — (fondly referred to by its victims as SMS) which, if I was being harsh, could also be known as TPE (The Perfect Excuse).

The media doesn't do anything to help metabolism's reputation; in fact, it plays on it. I once heard a radio advertisement claim having a particular mattress on your bed could help you lose weight in your sleep. The idea was that getting a restful, unbroken, eight hours' sleep was better for your metabolism which, in turn, would help you burn calories more efficiently. You have to say that was a good one, and I guess they had a point: at least when you are asleep you haven't got your hand in the cookie jar. But these bed retailers clearly know that we are so obsessed with our weight that we will try anything to lose it. We will even consider sleeping it off. Some people must think women are really, really stupid. It's probably, sadly, because we sometimes are.

I just seem to look at food and it goes straight on my hips. Now it's starting to wrap itself around my stomach too. Since I turned 30 it's got worse. I've put on 9kg in two years. My best friend weighs 55kg and seems to burn everything she eats, which makes me feel even worse. I go to spin and pump classes when I can but it makes no difference. I haven't even had kids yet. What will happen then? My friend says my metabolism may be faulty. Is she right? Or is she just being kind?
Faulty, 32

Dear Faulty,
I feel sorry for you. It's not easy having girlfriends like that, especially when you are both in the general vicinity of cake. Hopefully you have some other friends too. It's true that some people burn energy faster than others — but faulty metabolism? No. More like sad, confused, bewildered metabolism. I bet if we looked at your life we'd find some pretty irregular eating, and exercise and lifestyle patterns. Your metabolism has probably checked out of town. Or maybe you never really gave it a chance to work for you. The good news is that you can entice it back. It'd probably like to come home anyway.

Many women describe their metabolism as 'slow' or 'lazy', or inactive, the type that just doesn't burn calories or, if it does, it's burning slower than damp firewood. Our bodies use the energy we get from food at different rates. While some women appear to burn energy faster than others it's also true that these women never sit still — they are very active. (Often they are very, very anxious too, but that's another story for another book.) They usually say they 'burn' food as fast as they can eat it. The implication is that these blessed beings 'can eat whatever they like' but the fact is they don't eat that much in relation to the level of activity in their lives. Besides, they hardly sit still long enough to get the lid off the cake tin. Do you see the connection? Or should I be a little less subtle?

There are two fundamental truths about metabolism:

1.   Some people burn calories faster than others.
2.   But everyone burns calories.

Very, very few people have their metabolism working at its most effective rate. Most people (unconsciously) train their metabolism to slow down — even stop — from under-use. In the most basic terms, your metabolism works like a car; if you don't drive it, the battery goes flat. And no matter how much high-quality gas (in other words, low-fat food) you put in your body, it won't change shape when the battery is flat.

Perhaps even more common is our tendency to bombard our metabolism with so many inconsistent messages that it just packs up and goes to sit on a beach in Hawaii. Who can blame it? Think about your own eating/activity regime. Is it reliable and consistent? Or is it as unpredictable as a woman entering menopause? (Hold on, don't go touchy on me — that was a joke. And we should be able to laugh at ourselves no matter what life stage we are enduring/enjoying.)

Let me explain what I mean about unpredictability . . . One day you feed your body well and take no exercise. The next day you overeat then guilt forces you to run (okay, pant) up a mountain. The next day you eat nothing all day, have a few drinks at night and weave your way home in the early hours. The next day you sleep in till noon, don't feel like eating till six, and then shove a massive, fat-laden takeaway into your body. And then you jump on the scales and see that they have crept up a kilo or two. Despairing, you tell people that your metabolism is slow, that you are losing the battle with your weight. Come on. Under that sort of irregularity how on earth is your metabolism supposed to know what to do, how and when to burn energy? I'd give up too. If you are serious about losing weight, you have to retrain your metabolism so that it knows what to do — and when to do it. And the key to that is getting some consistency in your life around eating and physical activity.

Let's go back to the car thing. If that analogy's too masculine for you, let's make it a pink car. If you keep putting gas in your pink car it will go well for a long time. Then if you don't maintain it, clean the spark plugs, change the oil, it will start to stutter and bunny hop along the road and finally stop. You need to hook it up to jumper leads to get it going again. That's what happens with our bodies. They need a jump-start to get freed up and working again. Once your body is working efficiently, all you have to do is commit to putting the right amount of fuel into it — at the right time.

Cars are lucky really. When the petrol tank is full, we can't put any more gas in them. With our bodies we don't have that kind of gauge. Sure we might have that 'full' feeling, but that's only a thought isn't it? We still have to act on it — or, more importantly, not act on it. Wouldn't it be great if the precise moment that we had had enough food for our daily requirements, the body flashed red neon lights and put up the 'restaurant full' sign? Actually it would be frightening because the sign would probably go up before noon most days. But more of that later. For now, we have to focus on getting your body working efficiently again. Pass the jumper leads.

Here are some tips for jump-starting and maintaining a healthy metabolism:

Eat breakfast. Your metabolism needs a reason to get started every day. Breakfast is a call to action. If you don't eat in the morning, your metabolism will slow down and when you do eat your metabolism won't be able to deal with it effectively.

Aim to eat three meals a day. Your body needs a certain amount of energy each day to function and your metabolism needs something to work on. It's okay to skip the occasional meal but not if that means you are going to snack — and you should never skip breakfast. All you are doing if you skip breakfast is training your metabolism to work on nothing. So it will begin to run roughly and, eventually, it may spit the dummy altogether.

Increase your activity. Even if you only walk more, do anything that burns calories and gets your body doing some honest work. It stimulates your metabolism to work more quickly and evenly throughout the day.

Get your heart rate up with rigorous activity. Even better than the above because you are burning more calories **and** looking after your cardiovascular system. Five times a week is the optimum but anything is a good start (see chapter 8 on activity).

Eat at regular times. This helps to train your metabolism to work steadily for you.

Don't stop-start diet. It's like shock treatment for your metabolism. When you break the diet (which we both know you will) your metabolism will have to re-enter the workforce. And each time it will be less motivated and more reluctant to do so.

Metabolism and ageing

A lot of women ask about the effects of ageing on metabolism. Experts say that as you age your metabolism can slow by approximately 5 per cent per decade. But that 5 per cent is often better accounted for by the fact that you are 5 (or more) per cent less active than you were 10 years earlier. The answer is to keep moving and not to overeat. But that advice has nothing to do with age, has it?

STUFF TO DO: READ THIS (OR ELSE)

Being threatening is not my natural style but I feel obliged to offer you the best of what I know. If you've been dieting or thinking about dieting for years you need to do something to jolt your metabolism out of its slumber. And you need to start NOW.

So this is what you have to do. Put yourself on a tough eating regime for ONE WEEK starting from today. Not tomorrow. Or Monday. Okay, start Monday if you want to but make sure you do seven full days. Don't be stupid and starve — but don't be a wimp either.

Go back to the exercise you did in chapter 2 in which you identified all the weight-loss programmes you've tried. Pick the best one and do it for one week. Or go on one of those short-term body cleansing or detox programmes. It's not dangerous: your body will cope for a week. Quite honestly, it could probably do with a break. The precise nature of the plan is not important (although everyone with a weight-loss programme to sell will tell you it is). What's important is that you do it.

Hey wait — I hear you saying. This sounds awfully like a diet. Where's the fun in this? Before you start throwing things at me let me say this. It's not a diet because you already know what I think about diets unless you've been asleep reading this. It's simply a new way of behaving and it's what you have to do right away if you ever want your metabolism to work effectively for you. I'm asking you to do this for three reasons:

→ To make a change — you know you need to do things differently or you wouldn't have invested in yet another weight-loss book.
→ To wake up your body — get the metabolism back from its beach holiday. It needs to get a real job.
→ (Most of all) to make you commit to yourself. Because I like you even if you're not particularly fond of yourself.

Remember, it's only for a week.

If you don't have a plan of your own, here are some guidelines to help you:

→ Eat only three meals a day (because that is all you need).
→ Make these meals **small** ones. No super-sizing to compensate.
→ No snacks between meals.
→ No skipping breakfast.
→ Eat breakfast and your evening meal as early as possible each day.
→ Clean your teeth after your evening meal so that you know eating is over for the day.
→ Drink water. Cut way, way back on everything else.
→ Check in with me after one week.

Note: Buy a box of dry fat-free crackers and eat one every time you would normally have a snack. This will stop you eating unhealthily between meals. It will also show you how often you snack between snacks during the day, which will shock you. Which is what it's meant to do.

Now here's the bit where you'll really start to dislike me. But I don't mind: when you've stopped screaming, I'll still be here for you. When you've done it for one week, do it again. (It's more effective that way. I'm also testing your commitment.)

After two weeks, you can stop and go back to a less harsh regime. But be warned: it's time to do things differently. If you don't, then don't blame me if things stay the same for you. To make things easier for you I've written up a set of rules for eating and taking exercise, which are a summary of all the best ideas I've seen and heard from all the research and all the women I've worked with. If you're like me: the impatient and always-looking-to-break-the-rules type of person, skip straight to chapter 11, page 206. (Go on, the rest of you have a peep, too.) But then come back here because you have some more reading to do before I'm going to make you stick to that stuff.

Food for thought

Biological factors affect your weight. But not as much as you would like to think.

Your past sets up your relationship with food.

You don't have to stay in that old, tired relationship.

A new relationship is often way more fun.

Your metabolism probably gave up on you and went on the unemployment benefit years ago.

Stop the yo-yo eating and give your metabolism a chance to retrain and do some honest work. Now.

5 MY BUM WOULD LOOK BRILLIANT IF . . . I COULD LET GO OF MY PAST

'I just did not see myself in that [movie] world at all. You know, once a fat kid, always a fat kid. Because you always think that you just look a little bit wrong or a little bit different from everyone else.' *Kate Winslet, actor*

While our biology contributes to our weight, it is our environment that triggers overweight difficulties. Sometimes a past event has set up feelings of shame and disgust with our bodies; sometimes it's subtle (or not so subtle) pressure from families or peers; sometimes it's a single taunt or throwaway remark that spawns a lifetime of body image or weight problems. And always — always — there's society and the media's messages that slim is best, that slim gets the guy (or girl) and that, ultimately, slim equals happiness.

Let's talk briefly about the media because it gets such a hard time for putting the heat on women to be thin. It deserves some of what it gets because it began to set us up for weight issues 40 years ago. Before TV and the glossies women could only compare themselves with their friends, neighbours and a few thin-but-untouchable movie stars. Ever since we've had a whole lot of beautiful skinny women invade our lives through the media and **we just can't get away from them**. In the media's defence, it is just the messenger. It reflects society's beliefs about our bodies and weight and, dare I say it, our own often screwy feminine thinking. So 'fat' is depicted as miserable and 'skinny' as the ideal state. If you need confirmation of this, and I suspect you don't, check out all the 'before' and 'after' pictures in weight-loss advertisements and stories. These people always look utterly despairing before they lose weight — and outrageously delighted when they've done it. It's not just weight either: have you noticed how they save the flattering make-up, new hairdo and trendy clothes for the 'after' shots? Of course it's a marketing trick. But it still sets up a belief: **being thin equals happiness.** Be thin and you will have a wonderful life. Which would be really excellent if it was true. Unfortunately, that belief causes more misery than anything else because you don't suddenly become happy when you lose weight; you become paranoid. Suddenly it's not about whether you will regain the weight. It's about **when.**

Abuse and your weight

I'd never claim to adequately address abuse issues in a book on weight loss. That would undermine the seriousness of such events and experiences — and their impact on people's lives. But it would also be naive not to bring it up because there's an established link between past trauma and weight gain and/or inability to lose weight. So I'll just say this: if you have been sexually, physically or emotionally abused, either historically or recently, and it's affecting your capacity to live and function well please consider getting some professional help. It doesn't necessarily mean you need years of therapy but those experiences may be why you have struggled to make progress — not just with your weight but also in other areas of your life.

All forms of abuse have the potential to do some pretty nasty things to a woman's self-esteem and body image, which needs to be addressed, not just in terms of helping you lose weight but to help you lead a fuller more satisfying life. So please do it now. Why wait? You and your potential happiness have been in the holding pen for long enough.

In the beginning . . .

A woman's weight problems can often be tracked to things she couldn't control as a child or teenager such as name calling, teasing, bullying or social problems. Sometimes, as I've just touched on, there are more serious issues, such as sexual, physical or emotional abuse, familial or domestic violence or neglect. Weight-loss literature offers many stories of women who have lost weight, sometimes dramatically, once they have addressed problems in their past. In reality, this has little to do with their weight. It's about a woman gaining an understanding of why she is the way she is that allows her to move forward in all aspects of her life — including her physical appearance. I know of a woman who lost 18kg in just a few months with very little effort (although she was sensible about eating and activity) when she began to understand the impact of being raped in her early teens. She wasn't talking about her body when she said: 'I feel lighter'. Because she'd finally begun to accept herself and to let go of her trauma, and related beliefs, she was sure she wouldn't regain any weight, and so was I.

When did you first become conscious of your weight? As an adult? As a teenager? Or earlier? Women can usually identify that moment with pinpoint accuracy. And they can offer a surprising amount of detail about the event, circumstances or comment that started it.

When I was 11 years old a boy in the school playground called me 'blobby'. I can remember . . . I'd just got down off the monkey bars. I couldn't get his words out of my head. Even when I was 19 and pretty gorgeous (if I do say so myself) I still thought I was fat. Now I really am fat and I can't stop thinking of myself as 'blobby'. I think about my weight and dieting every day but I hardly ever do anything about it — it's like I've given up. I feel like I've been obsessed with my weight all my life and I wanna get off the train.
Blobby, 40

Dear What's-your-real-name-because-Blobby-doesn't-work-for-me,
Pretty gorgeous at 19, huh? I bet you still are. What you are not is weird. Or obsessed. But you are on a train — and it's standing

room only. Most of your friends and family are on the train too: weight-food-binge-diet-guilt-failure-give-up-start-again. But if you think it's bad for us, it's worse for our daughters. The poor kids have weight-obsessed mothers. Research tells us that mothers have a huge influence over the way young women think and behave in relation to food, diet and exercise. So you're right, it's time to get off the train. Not just for ourselves — but our kids.

Here are some other examples:

My mother made me go to Weight Watchers when I was 12. I did what I was told, I lost weight and my mother was happy. Ever since I've thought of losing weight as a way to get people to like me.

My family called me 'Duffy' because they said I was shaped like a plum duff pudding. And that's how I saw myself. [This came from an 81-year-old woman, proving that women's weight issues didn't just start 40 years ago when the media got hold of them.]

My dad used to slap my hands whenever I reached into the chip bowl. My three sisters were skinnier so they were allowed to have as many chips as they liked.

I was a very good dancer . . . my parents stood me in front of the mirror in my underwear and drew on me with a green marker pen to show the areas where I needed to lose weight.

My mother always told me 'boys don't like fat girls'.

A group of boys at school used to call me a 'fat pig'. It started after I rejected one of them. I can still hear their voices 'fat pig, fat pig'. The irony is that I wasn't even overweight back then.

The reason that people, and often people who love us, do and say these things doesn't matter much. You and I can't change them, but we can change you. The problem is that these comments or events may lead a woman to have distorted beliefs about her body and begin a cycle of body dissatisfaction that can last for life. These comments often mark the moment when a girl or young woman's weight slips into her consciousness. In reality, the physical self-consciousness probably started way before that. I mean it. Young girls haven't got a chance when it comes to separating out their looks and self-worth. Have you noticed people always commend little girls on the way they look: What a beautiful butterfly hair tie. Hey that's a pretty pink top. Gosh, what gorgeous wavy hair. Don't you look cute today?

Boys are more likely to get comments about school and their teacher and their age. Physical remarks tend to be about the truck logo on their T-shirt. Don't believe me? Conduct your own experiment by listening to people talk to kids and notice how early the conditioning starts. I was working with some four- and five-year-olds a few years back and as each of them came into the room I heard myself do the same thing: commenting on the girls' looks and asking the boys about their favourite subject. So I became determined not to do that. I started saying things like 'You look clever today', 'You're good at reading', 'I bet you can run fast'. I have no conclusive proof that this made any difference whatsoever but at least I didn't have to beat myself up for perpetuating the boys-will-be-boys and girls-should-be-pretty stereotype.

Even now I think it's better to compliment a person on who they are or what they've done than how they look. Don't get me wrong: I'm not above offering a genuine compliment about a woman's appearance (or receiving one if it's ever on offer) but it's much more likely to be about her shoes or her glasses or eyes or hair because those things don't relate to weight or body shape. And I think comments on personal interests, strengths or achievements are even better because they help to build our self-worth based on our unique personal attributes.

JESS'S STORY

I was at a young girl's tenth birthday party where the highlight was a game in which you dipped your face in a trough of whipped cream in search of a marshmallow. It was kind of cool if you didn't have to clean up the mess or wash the cream out of the clothes. Those who didn't — the kids — loved it. Except for one of them.

Jess was bigger than the other kids, taller, more physically developed, on the cusp of adolescence. She didn't launch into the game: instead, she hung on the fringes circumnavigating the cream, staring at it, being drawn towards it, finally lunging at it and, after, saying out loud: 'I wonder how many kilos that will put on me?'

Many of the women I work with tell me their body consciousness began even younger than Jess's, as early as seven years. What triggered it? Reports vary: a chance remark, a sudden awareness of their body, feeling left out of the group. It's different in every case but the legacy is the same: a belief that life would be better if you were thin, that people would like you more: that you'd fit in and be popular.

It also causes us to think that being thin is **hard work**, it's a battle we'll have to fight **all** of our lives. The sad part is that for many (maybe most) girls early childhood is no longer about riding a bike, climbing a tree or even playing with dolls. It's about looking hip and cool, wearing label-studded clothes and watching what you eat. Which has its place. But not when you are seven.

How do you feel about your body?

MOLLY'S STORY

Molly, 21, came to see me to get some help with panic attacks. When she got stressed, the panic would rise up on her so fast that her breath literally got stuck in her throat. She was a model client, always did her homework, was articulate and engaging, but when I encouraged her to go swimming to help her breathing and up her activity levels she refused as abruptly as a pony in a show-jumping round. Her sudden coldness was so out of character that I burst out laughing. I know it wasn't an appropriate time to laugh but I'm only a person remember. I mess up too sometimes.

'I'd never get into togs,' she said. '**Never!**' (As if I hadn't heard her the first time even though she'd yelled.)

Here was a young and gorgeous brunette with a hatred of her body that was at extreme odds with the way she looked. If I'd ever had a body like that I'd have had it on show at every (appropriate) opportunity. But an incident of sexual assault as an 11-year-old, followed by two abusive relationships, had left her with a distaste not just for her body but for herself. Breathing wasn't what she needed help with. Once we started in on her body (and self) image, she made rapid progress. Molly was last seen down at the pool. Okay, I made that bit up, but at our final session she promised me she'd go.

While Molly's story was her own, her mental picture of her body is common to many women. Really? you say. Then ask yourself this . . . How many women do you know who **like** their bodies to the point of not wanting to change anything about them. You know, if only I could lose a bit here, tone a bit there; nip, tuck, tighten, straighten, smooth, remove . . . the list goes on. Write your answer here. Notice that I haven't left a space for you to write. That's because I'm confident you don't need it, because you can't think of any. Can you? Even those you think should be happy with the way they look are not. I swear. It's a Western world phenomenon: female attractiveness has got inextricably bound up with physical appearance. Slim women are praised, applauded and perceived as being more competent and in control, which, at least some of the time, is total rubbish. Thin, glamorous and looking-totally-in-control women can be scary. And they can have problems too.

Perhaps we have much to learn from other cultures? I recall a TV documentary about women in a primitive tribe who wore pretty much nothing and seemed to have absolutely no hang-ups about their bodies. Their self-esteem seemed to hang on the number of strings of coloured beads they wore and how many children they had to the guy they shared with several other women. I admired their physical ease, even though it wouldn't work for me. If being attractive meant having 12 kids and a serial philandering partner then I'd be seriously happy having no looks at all. The point is, physical attractiveness means different things to different people. It's just that in the Western world it's way too closely correlated with the size of our bum.

So what is body image?

Your body image is not how you look. Your body image is how you think you look. And how you feel about the way you think you look.

Being dissatisfied with your body doesn't mean you are weird. It just means you're a woman. Being a little unhappy with your looks is okay until the point when it starts making you feel inadequate or it interferes with you getting on with your life. Even though women are often united in their negative feelings about their bodies, they are unique in the way these feelings originated and in what's keeping them going. That is why the one-size-fits-all approach to weight loss never works: you need a plan designed for **you.**

What is **your** body image? Now there's a question. Allow me to be a little presumptuous and assume you're reading this book because you're not thrilled with the way you look — and it bugs you to a greater or lesser extent. So what you need to do is unpack your own body image because this is what sets up, drives and maintains your efforts to lose weight. There are two key things to consider in assessing your body image:

1 How do you feel about your body right now? This tells us whether your concerns are negatively affecting you and your capacity to live fully.

2 What factors are maintaining those feelings — this is the most important because these are what keep us 'stuck' in our efforts to lose weight.

STUFF TO DO: YOUR BODY IMAGE

This exercise has two parts so take your time. Both parts are important but pay particular attention to the second because this will help you with what you absolutely have to know to make progress.

Part One: How do I feel about my body right now?
Are you excessively focused on your physical appearance? Are you doing things that prevent you from fully enjoying life? These questions aim to help you figure out which areas are of most concern to you and which you should target first.

In the past six weeks I have...	Sometimes	Often	Never
General body image			
Felt unhappy about my body			
Worried others will judge my body			
Felt disgusted with myself because of my shape			
Felt my body makes me unattractive			

My bum would look brilliant if . . .

Thought people were negatively focusing on my body			
Wanted desperately to lose weight			
Attempted to lose weight			
Sought reassurance about my shape from others			
Criticised my body (to myself or others)			
Felt embarrassed in sports clothing or summer clothes			
Self-assessment			
Checked my appearance in the mirror			
Focused on the body parts that worried me			
Weighed myself			
Measured myself			
Pinched or felt fat deposits or rolls			
Assessed my size in other ways			
Compared my body with others			
Avoidance			
Avoided looking in mirrors or glass windows			
Avoided swimming or other exercise that exposes shape			
Dressed in clothes that disguise shape			
Avoided being seen naked			

Avoided clothes shopping			
Avoided close physical contact because of my shape			
Turned down invitations to go out			
Hidden my shape from others			
Stayed away from social events			

Understanding your answers

Now take a look at the table. Again, your answers are not about keeping score. The idea is to identify the nature and extent of your distress with your body — and how much it interferes with the quality of your life. If you feel you are being held back or restricted, it's time to do something about it. Use your answers to work out your top priorities. We have to fully understand the problem before doing something about it. And we need to accept where we're at right now. The moment we fully accept ourselves is the moment we can begin to change.

The way we feel about our bodies is connected to deeper beliefs we have about physical appearance, either our own or more generally, about how we think women should look. Here are some of the common ones:

→ I'm not worthwhile when I'm fat.
→ I'm not loveable when I'm overweight.
→ I'm fat, ugly and useless.
→ I'm a disgusting person.
→ I have to lose weight to get approval.
→ I'll never find love when I'm so lumpy.
→ You have to be slim to be attractive.

It's likely some of these beliefs relate to you — or you have similar ones. Psychologists help people target these beliefs and replace them with healthier alternatives. We'll discuss this in more detail in chapter 7. But one of the best ways to do this in relation to weight loss is to change the way you do things in relation to eating and exercise because that gives you early encouragement. That's why dieting and exercise programmes can work initially — they make you feel as if you are taking charge and that makes you feel better. But the secret is to use strategies that can be implemented permanently. And the even bigger secret is to get other areas of your life under control and moving forward.

Part Two: What is maintaining my (negative) body image?

The key to dispelling your negative body image is to figure out specifically what is keeping it going. Psychology suggests lots of ways to do this and using a visual image is one of the best. Check out this diagram.

In the circle write down your main problem. Some examples include: I'm overweight; I hate my body; I can't lose weight. Then, also in the circle, add the main negative impact this problem is having on your life (you have to write the reason to give the statement more power). So you might add one of these statements: it stops me finding a partner; it wrecks my self-confidence; I feel like I have no energy; I avoid social activities because I don't want to be seen in public. (So in the circle you might have written this: I hate my body so I avoid going to social events. Or this: I'm fat and unattractive so I'll always be on my own.)

Then in each of the spaces provided around the circle write down the things that you think are contributing to your weight problems or your beliefs about your weight. It's important to come up with the reasons that are specific to **you** and your environment:

You might find you've written things like:

→ My flatmates are always eating junk food so I join in.
→ I eat because I've got nothing better to do.
→ My partner keeps criticising my weight.
→ I'm too lazy to cook proper meals.
→ Having to cook for my family means it's hard to cook and eat my own food.
→ I always snack in front of TV.
→ My only exercise is walking to the bus.

These are just examples, but you need to give this some thought because these are the things that you need to work on changing.

So what can I do about it?

We think we want to lose weight because we don't like the way we look. But it's not really that. It's that we don't like the way we feel about the way we look. If we felt okay about our bodies, none of this weight stuff would matter. I wouldn't write this book because you wouldn't read it. We would just let our bums trail behind us and get on with the business of living.

Hopefully you've already started to make changes by putting yourself on a tough eating regime for the next week. Now I want you to do one more small thing. Return to the exercise you just completed and consider all the things that have and are wrecking your best efforts to lose weight. Pick one you think you could do something about right now. Think of **one** practical thing you could do differently. Even if it's a very small thing. Note: If you are already cutting back your food intake choose something that relates more generally to your lifestyle.

Write it down. It's important to frame it positively (so talk about what you will do rather than what you won't) and give it a realistic timeframe.

Let's say you spend most evenings in front of TV and that's when you snack. You could choose an interest, say photography, that you've never put much time into. So you write: I'll spend the next two Wednesday evenings figuring out how to fully use my camera and digital software.

Maybe you decide you're way too inactive. So you write: I'll walk four flights of stairs once a day in my office building for the next five work days. Or: I'll go aqua-jogging with a friend on Wednesday night.

Now you have to do it. This is always the challenging bit. But if you've made the task small enough and the timeframe realistic you will achieve it. And the result? You'll have a sense of control and achievement **and** you'll be one week into forming a new habit, the first step in making lasting changes. Well done.

Changing your life (and bringing your weight along for the ride)

You can change. I know this because I've seen clients change their thinking and behaviour, and improve the quality of their lives. It's the philosophy on which much psychology is built and it works. But in order to change, you have to want to pretty badly. It's not a matter of squeezing your eyes tightly shut and whispering to your 85kg self: 'I really, really want to be a taut and toned 60kg.' That's called wishing, and wishing belongs in Disneyland. It's also called wasting your time.

Wanting something is one thing but it's next to useless if you don't do something about it. It's like itching. The best way to get rid of the itch is to scratch it. But if you're not prepared to scratch it then you've got to put up with the itch.

I don't doubt any woman's commitment to wanting to strip off those extra kilos in the same way I don't doubt other people's desires to be sober or rich. Desire is a valid first step. But desire, and even decision, without action is no use at all. It won't change much. If anything, it will make you unhappier because you will have widened the gap between what you are and what you want to be. The size of that gap dictates your unhappiness with your life — as well as your weight. And the more entrenched those personal tensions, the more miserable you are.

My aim is to close the gap between where you are and where you want to be. Not by lowering your expectations or aspirations, though. Oh no. By making some changes to where you are now.

ALI'S STORY

Here's another story about a friend. This particular woman threatened me with friendship withdrawal if I left her out and I wouldn't like that. So she's in. Let's call her Ali. Ali, now 41, had been one of those gorgeous teenagers that got the guy everyone wanted and married him and had four great kids, a nice house, a weekly cleaner, two holidays a year and a dog that didn't run away every time you opened the gate. You know, the perfect life. Except for the 13kg she'd piled on in the past two years, which had made her miserable. It knocked a big hole in her confidence, prompting her to join a walking group with mountain goat aspirations, which had made no difference at all. She was continuously on a diet, which she broke on a daily basis because, she said, she had no willpower.

One day we're having coffee and Ali's talking about how bored and miserable and screwed up (and fat) she is. It's because she does this so hilariously that I keep asking her to have coffee, even though it's mean because she gets all cranky that she can't have cake. (By the way, muffins are cakes. Just because they have celery or red onion in them doesn't make them a healthy option. So don't kid yourself. They're cakes. And often very big ones.) But back to Ali. After a while I say something like this that, even to my ears, sounds seriously odd.

'Your weight's got nothing to do with your weight.'

She looks at me like I've just told her she had a second head. So I go on to explain that the main weight problem women have is the extra mass between our ears. Also known as our brains.

'You're saying it's all in my head?' she says.

I nod and she just shakes her head like I haven't got a clue.

'I wish it was,' she says. 'A fat brain wouldn't stop me from doing up my jeans.'

See why I like her? However, like Ali, most women get it back to front. They believe that losing a few kilos will make them feel better and, with great rapidity, improve the quality of their lives. The truth is that a few kilos does stand between you and unbridled happiness. Actually it's more like 1.5kg, the weight of an average human brain. So your body is not the problem. It's the way you think and feel about your body. And guess who's in charge of that? Your mind. Your mind is what ruins your life, that's what defines your days and the sort of feelings you have about yourself. Not your body. If your body could get free of your mind it'd be out there eating whatever it wanted and having a ball.

The good news is you **can** change your mind. It's a woman's prerogative, as they say, and it's possible. You might be the product of your past; all that misery might be representing itself in those extra kilos around your waist or hips but whenever you're dwelling on it, remember this: everyone has a past. Everyone is potentially messed up by something, or someone, in their past. Look hard enough and you will find something. Something — or someone — other than you can be blamed. And you have two choices: you can either keep pointing the finger or find a way to let it go, move on and go after the kind of life you deserve.

Ali, like many women, blames herself constantly for being weak around food and exercise, for lacking willpower. I wish she wouldn't. **Willpower is a dated and unhelpful concept**. It's also possibly the most overused word in weight loss. Just as it is in addiction or in relation to any activity or habit we want to eliminate.

You don't fail to lose weight or regain weight because you lack willpower. You 'fail' because your mind and/or body do things without your permission. You simply haven't trained them to work together to produce the results.

What you must do

Most older weight-loss programmes focus solely on changing a person's behaviour, to reduce food and increase activity. A few more out-on-the-edge weight-loss programmes claim that the mind is the key so they'll deploy brain-reprogramming tricks to sort out your neural hardwiring. It's a nice idea, but anyone who thinks they can lose weight simply by thinking about it perhaps needs more help with delusional thinking than they do with their weight.

Newer approaches consider the role of both the mind and the body in weight loss. This is good because if we seriously want to lose weight and keep it off then we have to change both the way we think **and** the way we behave. At the same time. Trying to do one without the other is impossible. But that's still too limited. You have to do something else too; you have to do something more generally about the state of your life. You have to get your life to the point where it's meaningful to **you**. Then whether you lose weight or not won't matter so much. And as soon as it doesn't matter you have won the battle.

Food for thought

'Before' and 'after' weight-loss photos are con jobs. Not to mention digitally enhanced.

Unless you change your mindset, you won't be happy when you lose weight — you'll be paranoid.

Women are the same (in disliking their bodies).

Women are different (in where this dislike comes from and what maintains it).

Willpower is a term someone made up once to make us feel bad. Probably a man.

You have to change your thinking and behaviour and find a real reason to get up every morning.

Muffins are cakes. Often very big cakes.

6 MY BUM WOULD LOOK BRILLIANT IF . . . I DIDN'T LOVE FOOD

'For me it is not a cosmetic issue. It is an emotional issue. When my engine runs down, my drug of choice is food.' *Oprah Winfrey, media megastar*

I know you. At least, I know how you think. You've been thinking, obsessing, worrying about your weight for years. How many times have you thought about dieting, or planned one in your head; how many times have you tossed healthy items in the supermarket trolley in anticipation of making a 'fresh start'? How many times have you cooked and eaten healthily for a few days or even weeks only to have it all fall apart with a stressful event or in the general rush of life? How many times have you been 'bad' with food so have given up dieting for that day and resolved to start again tomorrow? Many times, right? So many that you can't count them — and you don't want to.

This is what you need to know: the only person obsessing about your weight is you. When I talk to my friends I am not thinking about their size and shape, unless there's evidence of a drastic change. Sure I notice in passing how they are looking but I am more likely to notice how harassed they are than whether they've gained 2kg. I am thinking about what's going on in their lives, having a laugh, trying to offer some support — and trying to get some for myself. If your friends are obsessing about your weight then they are not your friends. Ditto for your partner. Often they are doing it to make themselves, in some way, feel better. But that is not real friendship or companionship — and it's definitely not useful to you.

If your friend has a problem with your weight, then don't worry about your weight, worry about the quality of the friendship. That is unless they are concerned about health issues related to your weight such as diabetes, heart and lung disease, stroke or a cancer — don't blame them for wanting to look out for your health because they want you around for a lot longer. But there is a difference between caring about your health and nagging you about it. It is not your fault if they go on about your weight, just as it is not their fault if you die because of it.

Addicted to food?

My weight controls me. I think about it when I open my eyes and pretty much every minute of the day. I think about what I will eat, what I will buy and cook for dinner, and I get really stressed if I know I have to go out and there'll be lots of food on offer. Lots of temptation! I've done well on diets over the years but I always fall off the wagon. The trouble is that I just love food. I love the taste, the texture, I just love being around food. Food excites me. Am I addicted to food? Is there such a thing?
Addicted, 33

Dear Addicted,
Sorry (but happy really) to tell you this but food doesn't have the addictive properties of Class A drugs, cigarettes or even alcohol. So it's not like a physical fix: you won't start to sweat and shake if you don't get your daily cake. And if you do, you are scaring me. But you can be emotionally 'addicted' to food as a comforter or as a way of coping with stress or boredom. The trick is to figure out how you use food; what your emotional connection is to food. Once you know that you can get to work on it. The good news is that when you get your eating under control you will be able to have a little junk food every now and then without finding yourself back in the gutter clutching a takeaway bag.

Here's a test. How much do you think about your weight? How many times in a single day? Come on, be honest. Is it every time you put on your clothes (or take them off), every time you walk past a mirror or shop window? Actually, I'll tell you who doesn't — men. Well maybe a few men do, and I don't want to criticise them. But these are vain men, who you really wouldn't want to live with because they would hog all the mirror time.

Once you are obsessed with something it's very hard to let it go. That's why yo-yo dieting doesn't just fail, it's damaging for your mental health. It might sound a little dramatic but think about this: the more you focus on food — what to eat, when to eat, how much to eat, what not to eat — the more it will get into your head. Your weight, eating and food will come to dominate your thoughts, and all your waking moments — except for when you are not passionately engaged in something else. Maybe even then, if you worry about your weight when you are having sex.

Truly, every time your brain goes into free fall, instead of using it creatively to come up with ideas and solve problems, it will dwell on your weight, appearance, eating and **FOOD**. How on earth, when your thinking is like that, are you supposed to eat less — and keep doing so for the rest of your life? That's why those diets that call on you to eat tiny amounts of food all day long are not just ridiculous, they are playing with your head because they make you think about food **all the time.** When you are not eating one of those teeny-tiny meals, you are planning one, or buying one, or stashing one in your handbag, so you really haven't got a chance.

Why it's easier to give up smoking than food

People say they can't give up smoking cigarettes. Actually, they can because people can do anything they really want to do. (Okay, within limits. Expecting politicians to tell the whole truth, for example, would be unrealistic.) I believe people are endlessly capable: that's why I do this job. So when they say they can't quit smoking it's because they don't want it badly enough (yet) or they're not ready to try hard enough. They complain: 'Oh you don't understand addiction . . . I just can't help it.' They can help it. They just haven't quite got their desire to quit to the point where they're ready to back it with slow, steady action.

Now, here's a nasty little secret and one you won't want to hear. Losing weight can be tougher than giving up smoking. Smoking at least offers some incentive. You quit for a day you have a successful result: one day off. You quit for a week you feel some real success. You start to get some physical pay-offs too. No stale smell clinging to your clothes. No smoky breath. It doesn't take long for the chest to feel a little clearer too. But weight loss? Oh heck. One day of dieting and you just feel hungry. A few more days and you feel grumpy and tired. Trying to lose weight after one day feels like it's going to be for ever and it won't make any difference anyway. That's why most people quit before the first week is out.

Here's the difference:

- → You need to eat to live.
- → You don't need to smoke to live (quite the opposite, in fact).

So we have the ultimate justification for eating. We have to do it. It keeps us ALIVE. No one can deny the necessity of that. It can be particularly tough if you are the person in your world responsible for food: shopping decisions and cooking. But for all of us there are challenges because we can't cut out food altogether. That makes it a habit we have to half-break. And that makes it the toughest one of all.

Compulsive eating

Most women who believe they are addicted to food are actually compulsive eaters. So it's not the food itself that draws them in. It's their compulsion to eat it. Compulsive eating is just another name for uncontrolled eating, which can take many forms. The focus can range from the amount of food, the type of food and the speed and frequency at which it is eaten.

Compulsions are the behaviours that go with obsessive thoughts. So someone who fears germs (obsessive thought) might wash their hands 25 times a day (compulsive behaviour). Or someone who obsesses about home security might spend an hour checking doors, windows, appliances and light switches every time they leave the house. So while the problem presents as excessive washing or checking, it's driven by the thinking behind it. Compulsive eating is the result of obsessive thinking. And if you think about how many women obsess about their weight . . . well, we're all in trouble aren't we?

STUFF TO DO: ARE YOU A COMPULSIVE EATER?

Check out the list below to see where you fit. There's no need to rate yourself or tick any boxes because it won't make you feel good. Just have a think about whether you do any of the things below frequently, sometimes or never.

Signs of compulsive eating:
- → Dwelling obsessively on food.
- → Eating to relieve stress, worry, low mood or boredom.
- → Eating even when feeling full (or sick) from overeating.
- → Feeling nervous or down while eating.
- → Eating too fast.
- → Overeating regularly.
- → Seeking out particular (savoury or sweet) food.
- → Compelled to try what others have on their plate.
- → Eating in secret.
- → Hiding food.
- → Telling people that what you're eating is the meal you didn't have time for (when you did).
- → Can't stop at one treat item — have to keep eating until the packet/tin is gone.
- → Bingeing regularly or after a diet.
- → Hunger makes you feel edgy and uncomfortable.
- → Eating everything on your plate even when not hungry.
- → Nearly ripping someone's arm off if they touch what's on your plate.

Scoring:

So how did you do? You're a compulsive eater, right? Of course you are. You're a woman. Around 95 per cent of the female population are compulsive eaters to some extent. The other 5 per cent are so perfectly balanced around food we don't want to know them. Or they are kidding themselves.

Binge eating

We've talked about binge eating as a classified clinical disorder. Now let's look at it more broadly, as a problem for many women. Binge eating, in this sense, is probably best placed as a subset of compulsive eating. But we need to talk about it specifically because women are more likely to say 'I binge' than 'I eat compulsively'. So they are more likely to see their problem as one of bingeing rather than of a compulsion to eat. Bingeing, or excessive and/or uncontrolled eating, is most frequently associated with obesity or bulimic difficulties, both of which bring specific sets of clinical problems. But, as we noted earlier, just because a woman doesn't meet the criteria for an eating disorder doesn't negate her problems with bingeing, or eating too much in a short period. There are many, many variations on how, where, when and why women do this — and in how much it concerns them.

Although some research suggests bingeing is the top layer of a general pattern of overeating, it can also be a problem for women who otherwise eat normally (whatever normal is). While some women who binge are overweight, others are not.

Psychologically, the most important thing is to find out what the woman thinks about her eating pattern. If it's a problem for her, then it's a problem. The secret to cracking any problem psychologically is to explore the meaning of that problem to the person who's telling the story.

Women binge for four key reasons:

1 **Emotional distress.** Eating for reasons such as boredom, stress, anger, depression or anxiety frequently sets up patterns of over- or uncontrolled eating. The next chapter covers this in more detail. Also, women may binge as a reaction to difficulties, such as a relationship break-up, getting yelled at by the boss, or a financial or job loss.

2 **Constant dieting.** Continually watching what you eat, trying to obey strict dietary rules, and being really hard on yourself when you fail, sets up an all-or-nothing attitude to eating. So when you break the rules, even slightly, you tend to think 'what the heck' and hit the pantry or takeaway outlet.

3 **Intense hunger.** Also known as starvation. When you restrict your food intake drastically you become desperately hungry. No prizes for guessing why this drives you to overindulge in whatever food is close at hand.

4 **Feelings related to body weight and food.** Feeling down on your body, or yourself, or being filled with guilt, shame, anger, self-loathing — or feeling that controlling your food intake is futile — may prompt a binge.

What to do about it?

Now there's the million-dollar question. Hopefully you'll find the answers all the way through this book and, specifically, in this chapter and the next one. But the important thing to remember is that the triggers to eating, the reasons and the mechanism, the beliefs driving it and the things maintaining it are unique to YOU. You have to know yourself in order to manage it. So pay attention to yourself, and your own feelings, thoughts and behaviour, as you read this. Not those of your sister who's leaning over your shoulder.

The truth about 'healthy' eating

Healthy eating. Don't you hate that term? It's the overused twenty-first century politically correct term for dieting. There's only one worse way to say it: sensible eating. The idea of sensible eating feels to me like sensible shoes. The culinary equivalent of the shoes you wear when you are old and have bunions. Flat at heel and broad at toe; easy on the body, but no fun at all. What a bore: being old and having bunions should never rule out having fun.

But back to food. Everyone goes on and on about the difference between healthy eating and dieting and how dieting is **bad** and healthy eating is the **way to go**. People in the food industry pretend to do that because they want to spare us from the mental torture that goes with the idea of dieting. (And they needed a new way to pitch their worn out ideas.) They're trying to couch our food and weight obsession in nice, positive language. But it's just a spin job because healthy eating is as much of a con as dieting.

Check out the difference:

Dieting is about cutting back your food intake. That's not a bad thing because you do have to reduce your intake or at least adjust your intake/out-take balance if you want to lose weight. What's bad about dieting is the heavy focus it loads on what you eat and what you weigh.

Healthy eating doesn't bother too much with the idea of cutting back. It's more about having whatever the heck you want as long as you can feasibly say it's good for you. When used generally, it doesn't talk about proportion, amount, size; it says absolutely nothing about restraint. It says nothing about control. So, in effect, healthy eating is an umbrella term for doing absolutely nothing at all. Apart from making yourself feel good by making sure there are vegetables and fruit in the house.

What I'm trying to say . . .

Whoever came up with this clever descriptor is missing the point and being kind of insulting too. Any woman who has seriously tried to lose weight already has a good grasp of what kind of food to buy and eat. She knows that spinach is healthier than chocolate. She knows that grilled fish has fewer calories than fried chicken. She knows (hopefully) that weight loss is not so much about upping the spinach/fish intake as changing the ratio between what goes into the body and what goes out.

So give us a break: our problem is not about figuring out what to eat, it's about dealing with temptation, the utter magnetism of food.

BUT WAIT!

Before I get hate mail from everyone who believes fervently in healthy eating, let me say this: I'm not against a healthy food intake. I'm just warning you, if the only restraint you put on yourself when trying to lose weight is to 'eat healthily' then you will be in trouble. To shed weight you need to eat **less** food as well as healthier food. Temptation can't be conquered by good intentions. You have to get specific about what you do — and what you need to do — because being specific is the key to changing any behaviour.

So let's be specific. There are four things to consider in your eating behaviour:

1.   **When?** Your eating patterns
2.   **What?** Your choice of food
3.   **How?** Your style of eating
4.   **Why?** Your thoughts about food

Note: actually there are five things. Number 5 is Who you eat with (because that can really, really mess you up). But I'll have to write a book on relationships to fully cover that one.

Your eating behaviour

That your mind and body need to work together for lasting weight loss is well established, even though many weight-loss programmes still insist on making your body do all the work through diet and exercise. The reality is that you can't change your body (permanently) without changing your thinking. Trying to do one without the other is futile. It works in reverse too: if you change your thinking then your physical appearance will reflect new thoughts.

So which to change first: your thinking or your behaviour? Experts debate this with the same rigour as the chicken-or-the-egg question. However, in weight loss the answer is straightforward. You have to change the way you do things first. Changing your behaviour makes you feel as though you are taking charge and can provide some early incentive, which, as we've discussed, is why diets can be a useful starting point. The point is that our minds are very, very clever at going off and doing their own thing so it makes sense to use our bodies, or behaviour, to bring them into line.

STUFF TO DO: ANALYSING YOUR EATING

The first step in changing your behaviour is to have a realistic grip on the way you do things now. There are four parts to this exercise so allow yourself a little time. Maybe spread it over a couple of days because it's important. Not that the other exercises aren't, but this one is life changing. Actually it's weight changing. Which doesn't matter as much as changing your life but I know it's why you bought this book.

1. WHEN? Your eating patterns
Most of us eat randomly and spasmodically, even though we don't want to admit it. So try to be straight with yourself here. When do you eat? Is it on the run? Do you skip breakfast or lunch depending on how busy you are? Do you overload at dinner time? Scoff inappropriate snacks? Binge or overeat? Only eat when you are starving, then overdo it? Find yourself eating in front of the TV or in bed? Take a look at when you eat and see if there's any pattern to it or anything that triggers it. Identify your worst habit (including when you do it) and write it down below:

_____

_____

_____

_____

_____

Now come up with one thing you could do to change that behaviour:

_____

_____

_____

_____

Now you have to do that one thing. You have to start today. And do it again tomorrow. Do it seven times. So if your habit is a daily one you'll have it all done in a week. If it's a Tuesday-night-in-front-of-the-TV-thing then it may take longer. The jury is out on how long it takes to break a habit and instil a new one — even though lots of people will tell you they have the 'magic number'. Don't believe them because it depends largely on what's going on in your head. The key thing to remember is **the best way to change a behaviour is to replace it with something else.** So go to it.

2. WHAT? Your choice of food

We need to eat a broad range of food. A varied intake is good for us, provides balance and makes life more interesting. Weight-loss programmes that require you to eat the same thing day after day can be a good starting point but eventually you'll get bored. That's why you need a seriously good transition plan to ease you back into more 'normal' eating. If you want to lose weight then you can't eat food stuffed with fat or oil. You can't overdo the carbohydrates either. But you already know that and I'm not the food police. I would never say a particular food should be banned because that immediately makes us crave it.

Losing weight depends on you eating **less** food. If you can't afford your idea of healthy food, then just think about where and how you can reduce your intake. Don't use the high cost of fruit and vegetables as an excuse for not being able to lose weight. 'I can't afford it' is a modern catch-cry for everything. (Have you noticed how many of us say this and how often? Okay, we have to say it to our kids because they have a drip inserted in our wallets, but it's still a really boring thing to say.) Sometimes change is not just about change. Or how much money you have. It's about reduction. Most of us could halve the amount of food we eat daily and still be nutritionally sound. So check out the number of times you eat daily, the type of food you are eating and the size of your portions, which are almost always too big. And cut them down.

To lose weight you need to eat less food than you eat now.

Think of one way you could reduce your intake each day. Write it down below if you want to. But I'd much rather you did it than wrote about it.

....

....

....

....

3. HOW? Your eating style

How you eat is closely related to when you eat. But let's be clear on the difference. When you eat is all about timing. How you eat is about the precise nature of the way food ends up in your stomach.

So ask yourself these questions. Do you eat standing up as you race around the kitchen? Do you eat at a table? In front of the TV? At home or out? Do you mostly eat with family or friends or on your own? Do you eat fast and furiously or savour the taste of your food? Are you first finished or last? Is food just something to keep your energy levels up . . . or is it something you like to linger over while gossiping and relaxing?

Most of us can't claim rigid routines around our eating. Nor would we want to — variety and change makes life fun, if a little exhausting. But the random nature of the way we eat is a trap for our weight. Here are some tips:

Meals/eating (including appropriate snacks) should be planned when possible. This is so our heads can tell our bodies what's going on. Putting your eating on autopilot is asking for trouble.

Sit down to eat. If you don't have time then you had better re-read the earlier chapter on stress.

When you are eating, focus on eating. Eating in front of the TV is bad because you are consuming food without even really noticing what it is. So (potentially) you eat more than you need without fully enjoying it. Note: if you are eating with others it's good to talk to them. Don't be so food focused that you forget to do that. That would make you boring and a little odd.

Eat at the dining table. Just as bed is for sleeping (and sex), the table is the best place for eating (no comment on its use for sex). Families should aim to eat together whenever possible because it's a good place for bonding and learning table manners. Otherwise you might wake up one day and find your 14-year-old can't hold a knife and fork as well as a chimpanzee can. Which is kind of embarrassing. Trust me.

Be aware of what you're eating. See it. Taste it. Feel the texture of it. Food is much more fun that way and it helps you stop when you've had enough.

Aim to finish last. Not after everyone's gone home but you know what I mean. Eating fast and finishing first might satisfy your competitive nature, or quell your nerves, but it'll also tempt you into a second helping.

Go out to eat. Not all the time, obviously, but don't say no to all social invitations and/or freak out if someone invites you out for a meal. This is called fun. And I'd be unhappy if your difficulties with food stood in the way of that.

So what immediate change could you make to the way you eat? If you find this difficult think about how you could bring a little more regularity to your eating.

Start now, even if you can only manage it one day a week.

4. WHY? What's in your head

Why do you eat the way you do? I've read lots of books and articles that encourage you to eat food and think about food like a thin person. It's weird. Which thin person? And why should you? You may not even like this particular thin person so why should you copy her? You are yourself so you should think for yourself — not for someone you've never met, may not like, and who can probably eat whatever she wants no matter what's going on in her head.

If you are like most of us, it's probably fairly hard to identify your thought processes at any given time. Women's minds are complex things. That's what makes us so intriguing. It's also what scares the heck out of men. So I'm not going to ask you to do anything else right now. Just read the next chapter. Because it will help, I promise.

Using food weirdly

For all that we profess to know about the intricate properties of food it often gets dumbed down and dumped into the categories of 'good' or 'bad'. That's a bit strange because foods are a bit like people: highly individual and the good bits are often covered up by the not-so-good bits. Fish, for example, is doing okay on the health front until you dip it in batter and drop it in bubbling oil. Same for lettuce until someone with the full-cream Thousand Island dressing cuts loose. But the way we categorise food is less important than women's tendency to link the type of food they've eaten to their own behaviour. For example, when a woman says 'I've been good today' it's more likely to refer to having salad for lunch than cleaning the toilet. And 'I've been bad' is more likely to be about bingeing on thickcut chips than backing the car gently into a fence. This is actually really dumb because cleaning the toilet is a really good thing to do and backing the car gently into a fence is not. Still, if you want to be psychological about it, none of these acts needs to be labelled good or bad. They are just things that happened involving salads and toilets and chips and cars. Now I'm just sounding weird so I'll move on.

Food as a treat or a punishment

Do you ever use food as a treat or reward? I'm not talking about binge (or excessive/fast) eating. That's way more than a treat, no matter how well you spin it. I'm talking about allowing yourself to have a small amount of a favourite food. Like a Mars Bar at the end of a week of dieting, a brownie with your trim flat white or dinner at your favourite restaurant. Of course you have done this — everyone does — it's called **normal** behaviour. You see, in our crazy modern food environment the way we view food has changed. Going to McDonald's or getting a takeaway is not the treat it was ten years ago; fast food is built into our diets. Food is much more available too: Easter eggs, for example, can be bought all year round. Open all hours supermarkets and gas stations, vending machines and pay-as-you-go snack boxes mean we're within a heartbeat of a 'treat' day and night. So they're not really treats, are they? They're just food we grab and feel guilty about later.

What about using food as a punishment? I'm not talking about saying to yourself 'I've been bad so I'll deal with it by stuffing down a pizza.' It's more common to do it like this: 'I've been bad so I won't eat anything tomorrow.' That's called inversely punishing yourself with food. It's also called being a martyr. Which, sadly, is one of the hallmarks of being a woman. (See why I don't want men to read this? They don't need the ammunition.)

The trouble is that using food like this stands in the way of you making changes and, therefore, losing weight. So you have to break the cycle. Here's how:

Food as a treat. Ask yourself if eating this treat will really make you feel better. Actually, stupid question because it might, at least momentarily. But perceiving food as a 'treat' is a trap because it makes you think of food as forbidden — and once it's forbidden you **must have it**. You'll just hang out for the next treat and gradually the treats will run together to make up your normal daily intake. What you need to do is see food as just food: some of which you like, some you don't. So if you want to have a small amount of food you enjoy, just go ahead and have it. Not too often though. And call it food you like. Not a treat. Start to think about how else you could treat yourself: a new magazine or DVD, a bath with the door locked, a bunch of fresh flowers. I'm not being very creative here but you can: basically a treat can be anything you don't want to put in your mouth. So go to it.

Food as punishment. The idea of food as a punishment possibly started when you were a child and were sent to bed without dinner or made to choke down some vomit-inducing dish (that you were told your mother cooked with love) before being allowed dessert. Sigh. No wonder we get all messed up. Food should never be used as a punishment because it loads meaning onto something that should just be allowed to sit quietly on a plate and get on with its life. Also, you don't deserve it. You don't deserve any sort of punishment at all. Besides a day without eating anything tasty is not a good day. Why would we deliberately set out to have anything other than a good day? The trick to breaking the cycle is the same as above: see food as food, not as something with emotional strings attached.

The way we eat and the way we behave in relation to food offers many clues as to why we put on weight, carry excess and struggle to shift it. But it's not everything. Your mind and your body both have to be committed to the task in order to make lasting change. If either of them won't play the game, the relationship is doomed, along with your best efforts to lose weight.

Food for thought

Nearly all women are compulsive eaters. Only the degree separates us.

The only person obsessing about your weight is you.

Healthy eating is a useful term for people who want to do nothing at all.

You need to eat less food as well as healthy food.

The best way to change behaviour is to replace it with something else.

Food is food. Not a drug. Not a treat. And not an excuse for being a martyr.

You are in charge of your eating. Not some skinny woman you've never met.

7 MY BUM WOULD LOOK BRILLIANT IF . . . I DIDN'T EAT FOR COMFORT

'You need a balance in life between dealing with what's going on inside and not being so absorbed in yourself that it takes over.'
Nigella Lawson, food broadcaster and writer

Eating is such an emotional thing. Don't you wish we could stick to the evolutionary reason for eating: survival. It would save so much trouble, so much grief. But it'd be no fun at all. We'd miss out on one of life's great pleasures because food is so central to the way we work, play and live. We go out to eat, we have people over to eat, and we meet to eat: when we're having fun, food is often part of the scene. But the fun part of eating is not the troubled part. Women don't binge because they're happy even though actress Kirstie Alley, whose weight battles are the stuff of celebrity legend, says she does: 'When everything is going really well every day is like I'm at a birthday party.' I like her style but I still think if she was really happy with herself she'd be able to be at the party without eating all the cake.

Women's vulnerability to emotional and psychological problems, especially depression and anxiety, is well documented. Around one in four women will suffer from a clinically significant problem at some time in their lives but it is estimated that only 20–30 per cent of those who need help seek it. And for all those who are diagnosed and receive treatment, there are a whole lot more flying just below the distress radar. In an era when we Western world inhabitants are deemed to have it all, misery is common, dissatisfaction is endemic and our stress is killing us. And even though the answer can't be found in the fridge or the pantry, many of us still insist on looking there.

How emotions affect our weight

Women's happiness and satisfaction with their weight is clearly linked although some people are much more bothered by it than others. I'm not sure whether slimmer women are perceived as happier because they're not stressed about their weight, or that happy women don't have weight issues because they feel truly at peace with their lives. It doesn't really matter. And I certainly don't want to say that being overweight means you are unhappy and/or not on top of your game. That would be crazy as well as untrue. It would also be a very arrogant thing to say because plenty of larger women have their lives in much better shape than I have mine.

It's more useful to look at it the other way around. That is, there is often a link between women with ongoing weight problems and the amount of stress or sadness in their lives — and it may not be obvious even to them. Sometimes the problem is a current one; sometimes it's buried deep in the past. Sometimes it's something that a woman has forgotten, blocked, or tried to forget. Many cases of women who have been abused, like Jemma's over the page, demonstrate how they have used food to keep their femininity hidden or to make themselves unattractive to men. For these women the problem is maintained by the thinking these experiences have set up — because these beliefs rule our behaviour and, specifically, the way we eat. When they have had professional help to understand the impact of this trauma and how to move forward from it, they have lost weight. More importantly, they have staked a claim for their own fulfilment and enjoyment.

So think about it. Old hurt, resentment, fear and trauma may be the reason the tyre has settled around your waist or that the seams of the jeans two sizes larger than you want to wear are under pressure. That hurt and resentment is not your fault, but letting go of it is your responsibility.

JEMMA'S STORY

Jemma, 29, sought psychological treatment because she was struggling with anxiety and having panic attacks after losing her job in customer services. It turned out that her first boyfriend when she was 15 had abused her for three years and, shortly after getting out of that relationship, she married a physically and emotionally abusive man. After a few years she left him but withdrew into herself and, although she had a few friends, she did little outside work. She lived alone in a tiny studio. The sudden loss of her job of several years due to restructuring had triggered the panic attacks. Beyond the panic, her primary concern was her weight: she had dieted on and off for years but, ultimately, it had made no difference.

Jemma hated her looks; she never went to the gym because she didn't want to get changed or wear sports gear. And she avoided the beach all summer.

Not surprisingly, Jemma's self- and body image had been shaped by her experiences with men: first the abusive relationship she had not been able to escape from, then the violent husband who had made her feel ugly, guilty and ashamed. She had not had a relationship since. Without being aware of it, she had eaten excessively and dressed shapelessly to hide her body and to deflect the attention of men. Once she understood the impact of her experiences on herself — and her body — and began to direct some energy (and love) at herself, Jemma made rapid progress. She found a new more enjoyable job and even joined a Pilates studio, which was helping her not just get over her hatred of her body, but start to appreciate it. As for the panic attacks? Once she began doing the trauma work they just faded away.

'Comfort' eating

I'm a binge eater, especially chocolate. I binge when I'm down and stressed and bored — and lately I've been down and stressed and bored a lot. I can do a king-size block in one sitting. I've been back living at home for the past few months between flats. My mother drives me nuts. I've got a good career — I'm a policy analyst — but my current boss is the bitch from hell, making me work hours and hours of overtime every week. My whanau come to me with all their problems. But it's hard. They think I'm rich so they ask me for money. I'm over everything. Including my body. I'm getting fatter by the day.
Awhina, 31

Hey Awhina,
Slow down. That's a whole lot of stuff you've got going on there. No wonder you're into the food. On the bright side, at least a bar of chocolate doesn't want your money. It does, however, want your sanity and you have to do something. Misery, disappointment, worry, stress and boredom all contribute to weight gain. And when you are not feeling on top of life, your reaction may be to eat more — or simply to tap into the comforting properties of chocolate. The trouble is that when chocolate does what it's doing, you know it's not comforting at all. It's scary. It sounds like it's difficult with your whanau due to the expectations on you because you're successful. But what's the alternative? You're doing well and your success is something to be proud of. So break your life into bits — home, work, boss, whanau — see where the biggest difficulties lie and start making changes. One thing at a time. Because this much stress is not good for you at all.

All women have at one time or another used food for emotional reasons or what's often tagged 'comfort eating'; that is, reaching for the chocolate, pizza or cashew nuts when we're stressed, upset, overwhelmed or experiencing any other distressing feelings. Often it occurs in response to specific events such as trouble at work or a row with a partner. Women who have spent years dieting often fall victim to emotional eating because they lose the ability to read their bodies' signals. Dieting trains the body to ignore the physical signs of hunger. So instead of trusting your body to alert you as to when it's hungry, or full, you eat according to the 'rules' of your latest diet. This teaches you to eat with your mind or according to external cues and — presto — a pattern of comfort eating develops.

Women identify comfort eating with several key emotions. They're in no particular order but based on what I've seen I'd probably elevate boredom to somewhere near the top:

→   Misery and sadness
→   Disappointment
→   Loneliness and isolation
→   Stress or feeling overwhelmed
→   Anger and/or retaliation
→   Boredom

Comfort eating is, er, comforting. At least, the thought of it is. The problem is that the type of food we think of as an emotional balm is not helpful to our bodies, our weight or our health. Nor are the quantities we eat it in. I mean, unless you are a rabbit there's not much comfort in a stick of celery, or even a big bunch of celery. And even if you are a rabbit . . . well, we can't ask them, can we?

The other problem with comfort or emotional eating is psychological. So the reason we do it (to cope with the stressors of life) and the reason we think we do it (to make ourselves feel better) are two different things. Where it gets all messed up is that comfort eating doesn't help us cope or make us feel better; it makes us feel worse. **Guilty. Ashamed. Regretful. Sad. Weak. Worthless. Ugly.** So I'm not sure it's worth it. Actually I am sure — it's not.

Emotional eating disguised as 'hunger'

A lot of the time we kid ourselves by telling ourselves we're eating because we're hungry. No, we're ravenous. But what are we really starving for? Is the desire for food really driven by our base physiological need? Occasionally the answer is yes, although in a food-saturated environment there should be very few times in our lives when we're a heartbeat from starvation. Far more often our stomachs are completely innocent; the cravings are coming from our minds.

What is hunger?

Let's not be too academic about this. Hunger is the urge to eat. Hopefully the object in question is food. But whatever takes your fancy, I guess, as long as it's digestible and not poisonous. That we get hungry is not interesting, it's fact. The interesting bit is why we get hungry. Is it because we really need food? Is it because we see or smell food? Or do we want to change the way we feel?

These are the three key reasons we get hungry:

1 **Physical hunger** is a primal, physiological urge. It occurs when we don't have enough (or the expected amount) of food in our bodies; it usually comes on slowly and is felt physically (e.g. stomach rumbling, lightheadedness). Most of us feel hungry because we have eaten very little on a particular day, or eaten erratically, or been far more active than usual — so it's a real physical ache. Never mind that it's an ache we could quell simply by eating more regularly and without guilt.

2 **Opportunistic hunger** is a Western world phenomenon. It occurs when we are driving past a fast food outlet and the neon signs trigger a physiological urge to eat. Or the smoky aroma from the neighbour's barbecue has us drooling so we invite ourselves over (or I used to until they locked their gate). Intellectually, and to make ourselves feel better, we call this kind of eating an automatic response to food-related stimuli. In reality, it just makes us fat.

3 **Psychological hunger** is driven by our emotions and mental state. Often it comes on suddenly so we go from not thinking about food to feeling ravenous. It can be a craving or an urge, and it can lead to automatic, absent-minded and/or out-of-control eating. It's a hunger for something other than food. It's a hunger to feel different or better than we do. Whether we want to admit it or not, most Western world hunger is psychologically driven and disguised as something else:

→ Hunger for something interesting/meaningful to do = BOREDOM.
→ Hunger for love or companionship = LONELINESS.
→ Hunger for peace = STRESS.
→ Hunger for a better or different life = DISAPPOINTMENT.
→ Hunger for happiness = MISERY.

So why do you eat? Beyond what is necessary for your survival, of course. Be honest. Have a think about how you feel — and how you would like to feel. Because your answers will tell you where you should be directing more of your energy.

Coping with the 'tough stuff'

You've heard this before but psychologists always think you can't hear it enough. We are really boring like that. But it's okay to be boring and repetitive when you are 100 per cent sure that something is true. So let me roll it out again . . .

It's not what happens to us in life that matters, it's how we respond to it.

Our reactions to events, situations and people, laid one upon the other, determine the direction and quality of our lives. It's a big statement because it dumps the responsibility for your life on YOU. Oh heck. Most people would prefer to hide under the bed or blame someone else than take responsibility for themselves, their choices and actions. Not you though, huh? You're reading this book so I'm assuming you're ready to make some changes. That's why you impress me. And it's why I like and admire all my clients so much. It takes courage to shoulder your personal load and do something about improving your life. It's much easier to lie on your couch (not mine), hide under your blankey and blame everyone else for your misery than to step up to the plate and do something about it. But once you start to invest in yourself, you're on your way.

How do you respond?

How do you respond to stress, misery and disappointment? Do you go into meltdown in the face of difficulties? Or are you mellow and calm? Do you front up or go into hiding? Many women blame stress for their weight gain and they have a point, indirectly anyway. You don't put on weight only because you are worried or stressed. You put on weight because you eat more and/or do less because you are worried or stressed. A lot of the time you don't even realise you are doing it. Stress makes us react in ways that we would not otherwise. Sometimes it makes us tired or angry or depressed. Sometimes it keeps us in the house. Sometimes it makes us sick. Sometimes it makes us go out and do stupid things — with stupid people. Basically, it makes us forget to take good care of ourselves.

Some people carry their worries in extra kilos. There is often a link between women with ongoing weight problems and the amount of stress or sadness in their lives — and it may not be obvious even to them. Over time, the problem may become less about things that have happened and more about the beliefs they carry about themselves — because these beliefs rule our behaviour and, specifically, the way we eat. The trouble is that using cheesecake to chase down your worries won't make them disappear. It'll just help them stick to your bum, thighs and stomach. And give you eating-related guilt, shame and disgust to deal with as well.

The best thing to say about emotional or comfort eating is don't do it. Now I'm aware that this statement makes me sound horribly smug but before you start throwing things at me remember that I'm in your corner. I'm working for you. Trust me. (And if you must throw things at me please ensure they're tasty things in bite-size pieces.)

It's okay to feel sad sometimes, and afraid and lonely. But it's not okay to use food to compensate. A lot of times women say their overeating is automatic; an unintentional act. That the food has gone before they even realise it. That's a good theory but it's also a good excuse. You **do** have time to make a decision about what goes into your mouth. It's the period that begins when you move the food from its natural resting place and ends when it reaches your lips. Often it's not a very big amount of time but it is a window — it's enough time to make a choice.

What you eat is your responsibility, or if it's a problem for you then it's your problem. It's not the refrigerator or the cake tin or your friends or your family or the stress in your life. Those things might not make it easy but unless you are being strapped down and force-fed against your will then you are in charge of whatever goes into your mouth. Consider this example. Let's say you binge on a big tub of ice cream. Consider the steps you took from the moment you decided you wanted ice cream:

→ Put TV on pause
→ Climbed off the couch
→ Moved towards freezer
→ Opened freezer door
→ Removed ice cream
→ Grabbed spoon (bowl optional)
→ Returned to TV
→ Ate ice cream.

I know what you think happened. You put yourself on autopilot and suddenly the ice cream was being spooned between your lips. But if you look at the list you'll see eight actions. Each of those eight acts was something you could have chosen not to do, right? Don't beat yourself up; it's too late, the ice cream's long gone. Instead try to think about why you did it. Isolate the reason you went after the ice cream at that time. Think about how you could have responded differently to whatever you were thinking. Think about what you could do to stop that from happening again. One of the great things about being human is that there's always another way to look at something and there's always an alternative way to behave.

So, say you ate the ice cream because you felt grumpy because you'd had a bad day at work. That's fair. Sometimes life sucks. Sometimes you hate your job. Your boss may be impossible. But that's her problem. You've already taken her crap at work, no need to put on a couple of kilos for her as well. Think about the person who has to live with her and remember that it's **not you**. Perhaps it's a reason to be grateful — not grumpy?

So what to do instead?

The trick is not to just say **NO** to yourself when the urge to eat poorly strikes — that's too hard and, more importantly, it won't work. You'll still be heading for the kitchen. What you have to do is replace the eating with something else. It has to be something physical. It has to be something instant, easy and pleasant. There is no point dropping to your knees and scrubbing the floor every time you feel the urge to eat. Unless you just love scrubbing floors (and, if so, you need to check that you're in the right job). So take a look at your interests and activities outside the kitchen or wherever you prepare, cook and consume food. Is there something that you could pick up and do easily? Remember, it has to occupy your hands as well as your head.

Here's my three-step plan for countering the urge. You'll notice the first three letters spell the word **EAT** — I've done that on purpose. When you've got food on your mind you want something that pops into your head really, really fast.

Emotion. You feel hungry. You start thinking about what you're going to eat. You start moving in towards the kitchen. STOP! Before you allow yourself to eat anything, try to **identify which emotion** is making you want to eat. How are you feeling right now? Bored? Lonely? Stressed? Sad? Exhausted? Or are you on automatic pilot? Is this how you always feel when you want to eat or is it different? Stopping to identify your emotional trigger/s makes you aware of what you're doing. And as soon as you become aware you stop being emotional, **and** stop eating.

Ask. There are always a few seconds between craving/deciding to eat something and actually doing it — even if you have the corn chips ready on your lap. So before you actually allow the food to pass your lips . . . STOP! Ask yourself these three questions: **Do I really feel like this? Will I enjoy it? Will eating this make me feel good?** Let yourself become aware of how you will feel after stuffing down a packet of corn chips. You will probably feel bad. You will feel out of control and unhealthy and guilty. Is it really worth it?

Take action. Instead of eating, do the activity you have chosen to distract yourself at the precise moment you want to eat. One simple activity is enough. Remember that the activity has to be something physical — there's no point trying to picture yourself on a beach in your head because your body will be in the pantry doing whatever the heck it wants. Make sure the activity you are going to use to distract yourself from eating is ready to roll at a moment's notice. Don't tell yourself you are going to paint a canvas when you don't have a canvas, or even paint, in the house. Sorry, dumb example. I know you're not that stupid. Here's a tip though: if you have really naughty hands make sure they are both busy because you only need one of them to binge eat.

Changing your thinking

Your thinking underpins your response to people, events and situations. So if you are wrestling with the size of your bum, or any of your other body parts, it's a given that your thinking needs a tweak. We've talked about how difficult it is to get your head to bring your body on board too. Whatever's going on in your head has a pretty big influence on what you do. And when your body goes out to play it doesn't exactly leave your head at home with its nose in a good book. Although it'd be nice wouldn't it?

The value and potential benefits of changing the way you think are clear. But it's not easy. Your mind can play wicked tricks on you, which can be very distressing. I bet you've got plenty of your own examples. Think about the last time you obsessed over a man (please substitute woman if that's your preference). You constantly wondered what he was doing, who he was with, what his last words meant, what he really meant by that text message 'c u l8er' (when, if he was a man, that is what he meant and all he meant). You spent hours thinking about it, days maybe, when sadly you were probably just a fleeting sex-related thought in his day. And when you knew for sure he was not worth the trouble (like when he slept with someone else), you tried to let it go. Seemed almost impossible didn't it? Every time your brain got some down time, it would jerk back to him, dwell, obsess . . . So what's a gal to do?

There are just two reasons to change your thinking in regard to losing weight:

1 **To help you do things differently so you can lose weight.**
This is not rocket science. It's not even psychology. It's so fundamental that I'm not going to spend much time on it. Unless you do something differently in your efforts to lose weight your body will remain the same. So will your negative thoughts about it. This is the truth about women's thinking: even if we are only carrying a few extra kilos we think like the morbidly obese. We fret, we ponder, we stress. Men think they are built like Superman; we need to believe we are Wonder Woman — but with bigger clothes and smaller hair.

2 **To help you maintain any weight loss that you do achieve.**
Many women who diet hard and lose some weight continue to think as they have always done. That's a MISTAKE. There is no point in losing weight if you are still thinking like the woman you were a few months earlier. Not only will you begin to put weight on from the moment you have 'achieved' your goal, you will not enjoy your new status. You may not experience the full joy of your new look. You may live in FEAR until you put all the weight back on again and, when you do, you will be miserable about it. And so you will try again. While most women would say they hated this cycle, the reality is that they have come to expect it. And there is a certain comfort in knowing that this is the way it plays out.

So what works?

Psychology offers a whole raft of suggestions, theories and models for changing your thinking. Some of these demonstrate good outcomes with clinical disorders such as depression and anxiety. But some psychological concepts and techniques don't work well in weight loss. That's because they're impractical or, I believe, cause you to dwell on food or your body in unhelpful ways, or are difficult to use and interpret on your own.

These are the steps you have to take to change your thinking:

Be positive/optimistic. It's obvious, I know, but you can't lose/ manage your weight permanently if you believe you are going to fail. Because fail you eventually will. However, while optimism is helpful in all spheres of your life, on its own it won't work at all.

Change your behaviour. Reducing your food intake and increasing your activity will help kick-start new thinking. We've covered behavioural change so I'm assuming you've already started. Right?

Analyse and challenge your faulty thoughts and beliefs. You need to think differently about your body, eating and activity. This involves identifying, analysing and challenging your unhelpful thoughts and beliefs and replacing them with new ones. We'll consider this in more detail below.

Focus on goals or solutions. This orients you to what makes you feel good and what you want to achieve (rather than your frustrations with your weight, body and food). Of course you have to have some goals in order to be able to do this so we'll get to that later too.

Work on yourself, not your weight. Learning to view yourself as a person and treating yourself as well as you deserve to be treated is perhaps the biggest challenge of all.

Positive thinking and optimism

Many people think the answer to everything, including weight loss, lies in being more positive or optimistic. This is a fine theory but it is totally worthless to a woman who honestly believes she is fat. Why? Because her being 'fat' is her perception, her experience and her reality, so five minutes of forced optimism is not going to overcome 20 years of bitter experience related to her weight, eating and dieting. If anything, it will just make her positive all her negative self-beliefs were correct.

Look, I don't want to be negative about being positive. I just want to be realistic so you'll know I'm on your side. 'Positive thinking' was the brainchild of some of the pioneers of the self-help industry in the middle of last century. Some of these guys were, and still are, my heroes so I would never dump on them. Far from it. I admire anyone who puts a stake in the ground in terms of trying to figure out the best way to live — and they got to that place way before me. It's just that these early positive thinkers were average-sized men who popped on slippers and smoked pipes each night while their wives made balanced, home-cooked meals for them; they were not women desperately trying to lose weight while buckling under the stresses and strains of modern life.

Positive thinking has since been rebranded as optimism and this is best summed up as something you've heard a million times: optimists see the glass as half full, pessimists as half empty. Many people in my world see the glass as shattered too, but that's another story. Naturally, we all want to be optimists. This is because optimists have more fun, according to research (as if we needed research to figure that one out, but I guess the happiness scientists have to do something for their pay cheques). Apparently optimists also do better in their careers, are more likely to get the girl/guy and they live longer than pessimists. More importantly, though, they have a far better trip.

Here is the difference though. Wanting to be optimistic is smart. Telling people to be optimistic is stupid, especially when the person you are telling is female and has an entrenched belief that she is overweight. Your level of optimism is pegged to how you feel about yourself. The good news is that optimism, like self-esteem, can be developed, nurtured and increased.

It's all in your head

Before you can challenge your thinking you have to know what's going on in your head. That means you have to do three things:

- → Monitor your thoughts and beliefs.
- → Analyse what's going on.
- → Chase out of town the thoughts that are causing all the trouble and entice some new ones to move in.

While changing your thinking sounds straightforward, almost everyone struggles with it. I mean, have you ever tried to channel your thoughts positively, when negative thoughts are racing through your head? It's almost impossible because while you know you are dwelling on something unhealthy, there is almost a pleasure, or a comfort, in those thoughts. Recall a time when you got dumped by a lover, or had a fight with someone . . . think about how often you thought about him/her — not just because you couldn't help it, but because part of you **wanted** to think about them. Be honest: you wanted to recreate, relive, re-feel the heat of those interactions. So every time you had a free moment, your thoughts zipped back there.

Women are particularly good at this. Or should I say bad? Either way, you know what I mean: we think a lot, often way, way too much. Women have such capacity for lateral thought it frightens me. We can think of everything — often all at once. Our minds are like giant shopping malls: so much going on; so much colour, action, sophistication, style and rubbish under one roof. No wonder men are scared of us (especially when we're shopping). All sorts of studies suggest male and female brains are composed and wired up differently. While that may be true there may be a fairly hefty evolutionary component as well: maybe our brains are just like this because they have had to be since the beginning of time, or at least since kindergarten. We haven't got time to sit down and ponder a problem through five carefully laid out steps. We fling possibilities at it from all angles and hope one will stick. That's why women who are successful in business are often very successful. That lateral and flexible approach, when well applied, can be highly effective. So we should celebrate our thinking style, instead of beating ourselves up for it. Scattered thoughts are okay; they can underpin great achievement. The key to great thinking is not how we focus our thoughts, but how we apply and manage them.

The thing is . . .

Thoughts are just things. We can separate ourselves from them. We can observe them. Just because they sometimes fill up our heads doesn't mean they are correct; just because we believe something to be true doesn't mean it is — although we can play darn good tricks on ourselves sometimes. The thing to remember, though, is that thoughts are very powerful, they can be all controlling if we let them. So if we don't make some effort to manage our thinking, it will manage us.

You **do** have to create **new** thoughts around your body, food and physical activity. It's not easy because the thinking that goes with overeating or out of control eating is often as comforting as the food. But spending all day with your thoughts centred on food will create a food frenzy in your head so you will find it difficult to think about, or do, anything else. The trick is to assign food to its rightful place in your life — as fuel, simply something to keep your body going. Of course if you are a chef then you have more of a problem. The rest of us need to get a grip.

Monitoring your thoughts and beliefs

The first step in changing your thinking is to pin down the nature of your faulty thinking in relation to food and your body. **Thought records** are used in CBT to record and monitor thoughts and some of the newer weight-loss programmes also use them to track what's going on in your head in various situations. So far, so good. You do need to know what you're feeling and thinking before you can do anything about changing it. The idea is that once you have a record of your thoughts and beliefs about food, eating and your body, you can figure out where they are distorted, or ill-founded. Then you can replace them with sound alternatives that will serve you better.

This is what I **need** to say so the psychology profession won't beat up on me. The theory is good. Thought records can work well if you are committed and you make accurate and detailed records, interpret them properly and design behavioural experiments to support them.

But this is what I **want** to say with particular regard to weight loss: thought records are not much fun to keep, not very practical and quite hard to interpret and implement on your own. So say you are sitting on a bus snacking on M&Ms, or in a fashion store trying on clothes that all seem too tight, or in a bar sipping a wicked cream-based cocktail, do you really want to pull out your notebook and start writing down how you feel? This is not fun. It will not make you a magnet for other people. It may make you look like a geek. I wouldn't do this myself to lose weight so I'm not going to ask you to. It's possible, too, that writing down every thought you have in relation to food or your body will make you feel worse, especially when you don't have a psychologist or someone trained to help you challenge those thoughts.

Analysing your thoughts and beliefs

Our thinking becomes distorted whenever we are struggling in our lives and those negative or self-defeating thoughts lead to a range of distressing emotions. When we feel negative about something specific we often exaggerate them ('think the worst') or allow these feelings to spill over into our lives more generally. So, for example, a woman who doesn't have the partner she desperately wants may see a totally bleak future despite having a fantastic job, superb apartment, many friends and/or other great things going on. CBT pioneer Aaron Beck identified a series of 'logical thinking errors' that people make when they are depressed. However, we don't have to be depressed to think in illogical or self-defeating ways. Women who perceive themselves as overweight come up with a raft of damaging and self-critical thoughts. The following are examples of common thinking errors related to weight and body image.

See if you can identify your own common patterns:

Black and white thinking. Seeing things as good or bad and ignoring the middle ground. 'If I can't get my weight down to 6okg my life will be a total disaster.'

Overgeneralising. Drawing widespread negative conclusions on the basis of a single incident or limited evidence. 'This diet failed just like all the rest. Diets never work for me. I'm a failure with my weight and in my life.'

Filtering. Focusing selectively on the negative side of a situation while ignoring other relevant information. 'Jamie from work asked me on a date . . . he must have been turned down by other skinnier women in the office.'

Negative concluding. Assuming the worst when things go wrong. 'I haven't lost weight after two weeks of dieting so I'll never lose weight.'

Mind reading. Drawing negative conclusions by assuming that we know what others are thinking. 'I didn't get the promotion because I'm overweight and unattractive.'

Blaming. Blaming other people for our own difficulties. 'I would be able to lose weight if my family didn't expect me to cook big dinners every night.'

Labelling. Labelling ourselves with broad generalisations based on specific features, behaviours or experiences. 'I'm fat, ugly and a failure.'

Comparing. Rating yourself by comparing yourself with others. 'Everyone else at this party is more attractive than me.'

Challenging your thinking

Once you understand the most common patterns of your thinking you are better placed to come up with more rational thoughts and beliefs, and to find evidence to support these. So, for example, the woman above who knows she tends to filter information can stop and assess the situation more broadly (e.g. perhaps Jamie asked me on a date because we've sat next to each other for a few months and get on really well). Remember, just because you believe something to be true, doesn't mean that it is.

So try it yourself: identify your most common thinking pattern, isolate one of your own thoughts or beliefs, and come up with at least one piece of contrary evidence. Even women who say they are 'ugly' will be able to name one thing about their physical appearance that they like (or at least don't think is ugly) — if they push themselves.

Again, the theory behind this technique is sound. But even when women know their thoughts about their physical appearance are illogical, most still have trouble shifting them. That's why I don't spend a lot of time trying to get women who want to lose weight to change their thinking using forms and record sheets — and then talking about it. It's more useful, and you get quicker results, if you get women doing things that tap their strengths, give them a sense of achievement and provide evidence for new ways of thinking and behaviour. Besides, if weight loss is the goal, moving around beats sitting around any day.

Focus on solutions and/or goals

One of the best ways to break a cycle of negative thinking (about anything) is to have a reason to drag our thoughts outside ourselves and beyond our own dissatisfaction. Some psychologists might disagree but I don't think you can treat any clinical problem successfully without orienting the person to his/her future; without helping them to 'look up' so they start to believe there might be a reason to be excited about what lies ahead.

So next time you feel a burst of ill-feeling towards your body/weight, ask yourself this:

Does thinking the way I do (e.g. that I'm fat and a failure) **help me to feel good** (insert what makes you feel good here) **or achieve my goals** (insert your goals here)?

Focusing on goals or solutions turns your thinking towards what makes you feel good and what you want to achieve, rather than your frustrations with your weight, body and food. Asking yourself this question works because it immediately helps you to focus on what's more important: your reason for getting up each day. BUT the problem for most women is that they don't like the reason they have to get up and they don't have any goals — beyond, say, losing 15kg before summer. No one I know opens their eyes in the morning and says: 'Yahoo. I can't wait to get up because I want to restrict my food intake and exhaust myself at the gym.'

When women are unhappy with their bodies, the first thing they do is set a weight-related goal. Actually, it's the only thing. That's not smart behaviour because it pins success or achievement to losing weight. It also makes losing weight the **biggest** thing in their lives and we've already discussed the danger in that. If you've already begun to implant the visual image of your 'ideal' self in your head (see chapter 2), then you've done what you need to do in terms of a weight-related goal. What you now need to do is set goals **not** related to your weight because they will have far more impact on your happiness than your weight will. Not yet, though, I'm saving that piece of enlightenment for chapter 10. You have some other work to do first.

Working on yourself

This is one of the keys to changing your thinking but it doesn't need a special section because it's the major theme of the book. Your work on yourself began from the moment you bought this book or someone who loves you thrust it at you and, in the chapters that follow, we'll talk more about you, your self-esteem, your strengths, your relationships and your goals. The key to improving yourself and your life (not to mention stripping off a few kilos) is to know yourself. Then when you really understand who you are you can work out a plan to manage yourself (and your weight) and get on with the fun part of living.

Food for thought

Women don't binge because they are happy. Even though Kirstie Alley says she does.

The answers to our problems aren't hiding in the fridge.

Hunger for food often masks hunger for something else.

Comfort eating is never comforting.

Chocolate is more comforting than celery. Unless you are a rabbit.

Guys who weren't battling with their weight invented positive thinking.

Your mind and body need to be equally committed to their relationship for you to lose weight.

You only need one hand to binge eat.

8 MY BUM WOULD LOOK BRILLIANT IF . . . I COULD MOTIVATE MYSELF TO EXERCISE

'It's impossible to walk rapidly and be unhappy.' *Mother Teresa, humanitarian*

TRACEY'S STORY

Tracey came to see me one day after breaking up with her cheating (and married) boyfriend. She was crying all the time, chewing her nails down to bleeding and had started going to the gym twice a day. She was in her mid-30s, tall, blonde, curvaceous, fun and would probably have an option on another boyfriend within minutes of leaving my office. But these are not things I ever say out loud. I actually say very little initially because that's the way it's supposed to be.

'You know the worst thing about all this,' she sobbed, after a few minutes of dumping on her ex. 'I'm going to put on weight.'

Tracey went on to describe a history of fluctuating weight difficulties. She always hit the gym hard when she started a new relationship (because she wanted to look good) or when a relationship ended (because she didn't want to look bad). She always stayed at it for two to three months and always lost up to seven kilos (yes, it was that precise), then gave up and did nothing. Her weight always crept up again plus a couple of extra kilos as if, she said, to teach her a lesson. Tracey had done the maths: six more boyfriends and she'd be an obesity statistic. It depressed her even more than the loss of Mr Wrong.

I never like this trend.

Tracey's certainty about the consequences for her body of this breakup meant it was probably going to happen. Not only did this not-so-great guy have control of her heart. He also had control of her weight — and her self-image. As had other guys before him. Men don't need or deserve this kind of power over any woman.

The 'mind and body' thing

Tracey's story is in here to further illustrate the link between mind and body in weight management. When one spins out of control, it takes the other with it. Tracey demonstrated a very clear pattern of falling off the gym wagon within months and a belief that this meant she would put on weight. That she allowed men to dictate her gym regime was even more dangerous. As we've discussed, the mind and body need to work in harmony to achieve peak performance in any area of your life.

I first heard this theory in a physical education lecture when I was 17 and it seemed like the most sensible thing I'd ever heard: mind and body working together to improve a person's quality of life. Of course, it wasn't a new idea. The ancient Greek philosophers Aristotle and Plato were on to it 2500 years before us. Okay, they weren't thinking about weight loss back then but I suspect that was only because they were men. They no doubt thought they looked fabulous wearing nothing but a strategically placed fig leaf. (Some things never change I guess.) And, in those days, they had time to think. They probably didn't have to work 50 hours a week and keep the relationship afloat while trying to slip into a size-10 fig leaf. Sigh. Wouldn't it be lovely to study the meaning of life from the shade of an ancient olive tree? Not while standing on the side of a soccer pitch or driving to Brownies, or trying to have sex with your partner of nine years when you would really rather be watching soaps on television or stroking the dog.

But this section is about exercise so let's stick to that.

Specifically, let's talk about the word itself: **exercise**. It's an old-fashioned, outmoded term and the very mention of it is enough to send most of us screaming in the direction of the nearest sofa. It makes me think of shivering through high school physical education classes where the teacher barked out orders and we spent 40 minutes wearing ugly, baggy shorts doing something boring and absolutely irrelevant to the rest of our lives. The trouble is that while we were so busy being bored we missed the one really useful lesson that our despairing teachers were probably trying to pass on. Or a habit they were trying to get us to pick up — that is the habit of taking **regular physical activity**. Not so much to 'do' a sport but to see the benefits of keeping the body moving. What they should have told us was that this habit was essential to our happiness — if not at that moment, then later in life. Actually, they should have slapped us in the face with it. Not that we'd have listened because we were too busy thinking about developing other habits behind the bike sheds that would bring no health benefits at all.

What we needed to know then (and still do) is that engaging in regular physical activity could:

- → Improve our psychological health.
- → Give us more energy.
- → Promote a more positive and cheerful outlook.
- → Help us cope with stress and tough times.
- → Protect us from physical health problems later in life, such as cancers, stroke, heart and lung disease, Type II diabetes.
- → Open up social opportunities and fun.
- → Help maintain a healthy weight and set benchmarks for our future weight.
- → Attract boys or girls; no clear link but I put it in because this one might have jolted our attention.

I bet those teachers really tried. But we stood there in our shorts, missed the one lesson they were throwing at us for free, and thought about the big stuff like some smelly, hairy, pimply adolescent and what was happening at the weekend.

The result was that most of us failed to develop good habits around activity back when we should have. And so, now, when we know we should (and must) indulge in activity for the sake of our weight, if nothing else, it doesn't feel like a natural part of our lives. It feels like a most unwelcome addition, something that we have to do in order to at least maintain a body shape that we are already desperately unhappy with.

The point of all this is to say that if you force yourself to exercise you will:

→ Hate it
→ Avoid it
→ Snatch at the first excuse to stop doing it.

Think about the last time you committed to some sort of 'exercise programme'. Did it go like this? A **big** effort for a few days, or even weeks. Then at the first hint of rain, the first late night, the first niggling injury, you grabbed the chance to give it a miss, and then you skipped another day, then another, and before you knew it the gym membership was wasted and it was just money you could have spent on shoes.

That's why I never insist on 'formal' exercise to any woman who wants to lose weight. Don't get me wrong — if you are a regular gym/ Pilates bunny or play sports often or love hiking up mountains in your spare time, that's fantastic. You are an example to the rest of us. But just because we admire you doesn't mean we want to copy you. I have several friends who are regulars at the gym or Pilates classes; although I've given it a try, I don't feel quite the same level of devotion. What is only fair to say, though, is that gyms are much better places to be than they were in the 80s and 90s: the range of classes means there really is something to suit everyone, young and old, from dance to yoga to weights to boxing to cycling (spin classes). People in tight clothes no longer leap around in front of mirrors — well, a few do but you can generally get away from them. And there are specialist women's facilities if you want to be spared from all that testosterone. It's still a personal thing, however. Modern exercise classes spook me slightly because in some of them you need a degree in coordination to do the required moves. I make a fool of myself often enough, I don't need to top it up at the gym. And although I think gyms are a fine idea for some people, and particularly in winter or unpredictable climates, part of the joy I get from being active, when I am, is being outside.

In reality, the women who like doing that seriously energetic stuff are already doing it. Most of us are more mortal than that. Our attempts at formal exercise are destined to be a stop-start thing that will play havoc with our attempts at weight loss and the kick-start we are trying to give our poor, confused metabolism. Stop-start exercise can almost be worse than doing nothing at all because it's so confusing for our bodies, as well as depressing for our minds.

But wait. This is not about me giving you a reason to avoid physical activity for the rest of your natural life. You absolutely have to be active if you are going to have any shot at all of losing or maintaining your weight. And you have to make sure that your output of energy is greater than (or at the very least equal to) your food intake. The other available ratio is a disaster. Because, barring nasty illness or a low-budget trip through India, you won't ever lose weight. You will stay the same. Or get bigger. Faster. And I know you'd hate that.

STUFF TO DO: PHYSICAL ACTIVITY RECORDS

You may recall what I said about food records and women's well-intentioned propensity to lie. That's what happens when you are asked to record your food consumption. For some reason, it's not the same with activity. We don't lie about our efforts at physical exertion. If asked to, we would write down everything we have vaguely done in terms of being active and, this time, our memories are surprisingly accurate.

That's because we are **proud** of being active in a way we are not proud of what we eat.

So consider your activity levels over a week. For most people, it's quite random: no week will look the same. What do you do to raise the heart rate, get outside, move the body? Walk/run to the bus, walk the dog, swim, play touch, play in the park with the kids, mow the lawn, vacuum the house, wash the windows . . .

I'm not going to get you to write it down. Not because I don't trust you this time, but because it's a really boring thing to do. And also (this one is more important) because it's impossible. That's right, it's just not possible to distinguish between what is activity and what is not because . . .

Everything is activity.

Okay, lying completely inert on the sofa or in bed doesn't count. But everything else does. If you amble to the bus, it counts. If you walk from the car to the coffee outlet to grab your latte, it counts. If you get the washing off the line, it counts. If you plant some herbs, it counts. If you have sex, it counts (as long as you make a vague attempt at active participation). Truly, the only way of distinguishing between activities is by their level of **intensity**. And, barring involvement in an Olympic training programme, all of us can do **more** than we are doing now.

Physical activity makes us feel good. And you know why? I'm not talking about the physical endorphin rush that is supposed to be your reward for a workout. I have never felt that in the way you're supposed to feel it. Or maybe it's just that I've never recognised it because I've been too tired. No, the real reason it makes us feel good is that we've gotten off our bums and done something.

Exercise 'addiction'

Exercise addiction is one more of the hundreds of things the modern woman is supposed to worry about. I don't know about you but the idea of being addicted to exercise makes me laugh. I know a few women become gym junkies or run/workout excessively but this book is not for them. Some women keep going to the gym regularly because they know how hard it would be to start again if they stopped. They are smart, but they are also quite rare. Most of us are in about as much danger of becoming addicted to exercise as we are of sprouting wings and flying. In other words, it's **not** going to happen. The trick is to do something you enjoy, make it fun or social or make it part of something else. There is no such thing as bad activity, except the exercise that involves raising the arm from the plate to the mouth. But you already know that.

Often weight gain happens when you suddenly **stop** exercising. Look at retired athletes. A rare few stay svelte and toned, but it seems to take most of them a lot of hard work. It's because they haven't completely adjusted to life after sport. They get jittery, unhappy and hard to live with. Injury can do the same thing. Any sudden change in your input/ output ratio throws the body into chaos and often your head too because feelings of guilt and panic rise to the surface. Your body screams 'what's going on' and closes down operation. You have to use it or you will lose it very fast.

STUFF TO DO: RATE YOURSELF — HOW ACTIVE ARE YOU?

This exercise is not a quiz or numbers game. It's just a means of getting you to think about the amount of physical activity you do. And because this can change so markedly over time, think about your level of activity over the past three to four weeks.

1. If you do (almost) nothing . . .

No one does nothing unless they are confined to bed. That's why I put 'almost' in. But lots and lots of women do only the bare amount of what is required to get through the day. If this is you, you are relatively lucky (as well as very unhealthy) because it will be very easy to increase your activity levels. Even five minutes a day is a step forward. Not only will it get you started, it will give you a sense that you are doing something about your weight and your health. If your lifestyle makes even basic activity difficult then look for opportunities to build activity into your day: e.g. walk faster, shop faster, do things around the house faster, walk or bike to work, leave the staffroom behind during your lunch break, get active with the kids — concentrate on putting more energy into the things you already do.

2. If you exercise erratically . . .

This is better than nothing, so keep doing what you can but recognise that this is still awfully confusing for your body. Aim to do some sort of physical activity (that extends you) three times a week and stick to regular times if you can. Five bursts of activity is even better, and the amount recommended by health and medical experts. And activity that gets your heart rate up is best of all. You should be taking every opportunity in your day to be more active, so be alert.

3. If you work out all the time . . .

I'm surprised you are reading this book. If you really are doing this and still having problems with your weight — then either you have some medical barriers in the way **or** you are eating too much. Go and see your GP. And then if there are no organic problems you need to do an honest assessment of what you are eating, then cut it down.

Pushing your body harder

Many women believe that strenuous workouts are the key to weight loss. That's generally because any successes they have had with their weight have been at times when they have been challenging or pushing themselves hard physically. So they come to see exercise as THE SOLUTION. It's misleading, though, because you can't simply sweat yourself thin. Even the toughest exercise regime — if that's all you do — won't solve your weight problems. Getting on top of the whole food thing is more important, as is looking more broadly at your life.

Obviously, too, 'strenuous' means different things to different people. What may be an afternoon stroll up a hill for you might leave me gasping on the front porch and plotting to terminate our relationship. The reality is that to get health gains (cardiovascular, respiratory and weight management) you need to extend yourself aerobically (using more oxygen than you usually do without over-stressing your lungs) and/or anaerobically (going into oxygen debt). You need to get your heart rate up. It's good to sweat.

So think about your favourite activities: how difficult are they for YOU? Rate them on a scale from EASY to EVEREST-LIKE? Are you extending yourself enough? Often enough? Then, at least some of the time, try to push yourself a little harder.

Activity traps to watch out for:

➜ You may feel hungrier if you've just started an exercise programme. **Be ready.**

➜ You may believe you can eat more because you've countered it with a tough workout. **Be cautious.**

➜ You may act on the above belief. **Be sensible.**

➜ When you stop working out (and nearly all of us do at some stage) you'll be vulnerable to weight gain because your intake/ output ratio has changed abruptly. **Be smart.**

Going to the gym, doing Pilates/dance/yoga/martial arts, running or cycling are great forms of activity. **If** you keep them up. If you don't, you make maintaining a steady weight tougher and when you stop you are setting yourself up for an awfully big backward step. It is as much of a yo-yo effect as dieting. What are the chances of you at least temporarily stopping going to the gym? For most of us it's fairly high. How do you think gyms and health clubs make money? It's not from new customers, it's from repeat business. And I don't blame them at all, they've simply figured out the way humans operate. The reality is that gyms and health clubs have more sophisticated equipment and classes than they used to; the options are more diverse and exciting, and the clothing varies from season to season but it takes the same level of commitment it always took. **You** still have to walk through the door. **You** still have to do the work.

Weight training in weight loss

So what's the role of pumping iron in weight loss? I used to believe lifting weights was very unhelpful because it simply consolidated fat deposits but I've had to update my thinking. Lighter weights used in high repetitions, such as in pump classes, burn a lot of energy so can be very useful in weight loss. There are psychological benefits too: using weights can make you feel stronger and more capable. This is especially helpful for bigger women who may feel uneasy in the world of physical activity: these women are often very strong because they've been constantly carrying a lot of body weight, so it can give them quite a kick to see how much they can lift. Also, to put your weights back on a stack after a pump class — instead of carrying it on your body — can be highly motivating. Here's a warning though: pumping iron on its own won't bring you closer to your weight-loss dreams. You have to mix it up with aerobic and/or anaerobic activity for best results.

STUFF TO DO: GETTING MORE PHYSICAL

We're going to increase your activity. Actually, I'm not. You are.

Set yourself a goal. Make it easy. The aim is to have you succeed. Doing **one** new thing each day will increase your activity levels over what you are doing now. It might be walking a couple of flights of stairs, running to the bus or the cookie stand (not ideal, obviously, but you see my point), walking around the park on your way home instead of through it, etc. These are very easy activities and that's deliberate. The tougher — the more you raise your heart rate — the better. But the minute you get that obligation to exercise formally in place, it suddenly feels **hard**.

Fine, if you love the gym and while reading this you feel the sudden urge to get back there, but guard against taking up an activity that you are bound to quit. It's much better to start to build (enjoyable) activity into your day so you begin to lead a more active lifestyle that you will be able to maintain. It's far tougher to quit an active lifestyle than it is a gym membership. And it's much easier to convince yourself that it's fun.

So what could you do right now to be more active? All of us can add a five-minute walk or a flight of stairs to our day. It's just a matter of spending 30 seconds to think of a way to do it.

Write down three things that you could do immediately to increase your daily activity. Be creative. And you do have to write it down this time. Writing down what you plan to do is much better than writing down what you've already done because it's a call to action. Anyone who's been down the diet route knows that decision and commitment without action are next to useless.

1. _____

_____

2. _____

_____

3. _____

_____

Struggling to think of anything? Come on, try harder. Because if there is absolutely no opportunity to increase your activity levels, not a single place in your week to add anything, then you are either one of the aforementioned Olympic athletes (who should be doing something other than reading this book) or you are in trouble. You need to have a look at your lifestyle. It must be crazy. Check your stress levels too. **Because something needs to change.**

'Me' time

I think you've got the idea by now that I dislike 'formal' exercise. I liked team sports when I was younger but I'm a bit wary of the increased risk of injury these days. I think it's got something to do with the thought of trying to get the bus to work while on crutches. Other obvious choices like swimming, biking, or going regularly to an exercise class have never been my thing, although I'm happy to have my arm twisted when it comes to trying new things. I do walk a bit, though, and occasionally I'll up the ante and run between lamp posts but only until someone I know sees me and laughs.

I'm aware that this makes me sound incredibly lazy but it also makes me real. I can't help it if I would rather spend my free time reading a book, lying in a deck chair or hanging out with my friends. I could pretend otherwise just to make myself sound credible in the world of health and fitness and weight loss but I'd just be a fraud. I want to be healthy but I really don't like that 'working out' stuff. That's why you won't find a picture of me in here wearing a muscle-back singlet and showing off my taut body parts. I don't have any of those (taut body parts, not singlets) because I don't do what it takes to get them. And, sadly, even if I did workout hard my body probably wouldn't play the muscle game.

There is one thing that does get me active though. My friends. Whenever my friends want me to do something active I will. (Or at least I might; let's not overdo it.) I'd probably do it though because it would not be me against the weight machine or treadmill. It would be me taking the chance to get the goss and have a laugh. And suddenly exercise would feel meaningful for me.

Read this. Even if all the rest is boring you. It's really important because it's another one of the differences between men and women in weight loss.

For women there are only three really meaningful reasons to get active (other than all the health benefits, which we fully appreciate but we've heard a million times):

1 To get some precious time to yourself.

2 To see your friends in a social context that is better for you than having dinner or drinking wine (you can always save these activities for the evening).

3 To make you feel good about yourself. I guarantee you will prefer the weight you don't lose if you feel you are doing something that's good for your body.

So when you choose an activity, and are looking for motivation, make sure it meets at least one of the above criteria. If it fits all three, then you know you are on to a winner — and you should keep at it.

Oprah, personal trainers and other stuff

We've mentioned celebrities a few times already so I hope you're not getting sick of them. But celebrities are useful here because they show us how hard it is to lose weight even when you are really, really rich. In fact, it is probably better to be poor and overweight than rich and overweight because at least when you are poor you can tell yourself that money would help.

Take Oprah, for example, who's so rich that she can hire a personal anything but her battles with her weight over the years show us just how mortal — and vulnerable — she is. It must be hideous to play out your weight struggles on such a public stage: every time Oprah's weight blows out the world's media swoop on it and she has to step up and explain it. She's had personal chefs, fitness trainers, weight-loss gurus and probably even psychologists — and her weight is still the Great Challenge of her Life. When you're struggling to pay the grocery bill (as well as lose weight) Oprah's story sounds pretty depressing. But it shouldn't be; it should be uplifting — because it shows us that money isn't the bottom line in weight loss. Not at all. Oprah's struggle has never been about paying for help; it's much more personal than that. Sure, we can kid ourselves that we'd lose so much more weight if we could afford to buy in the right help. But it probably wouldn't make any difference at all. I actually think Oprah's done well in the face of all that temptation: if I moved into her house I can assure you my life wouldn't be about restraint. Oh no. Show me to the pool. And pass the cocktails.

A lot of women pin their hopes on hiring a personal trainer down at the gym. But you need to be careful about who you trust with your weight. These trainers are often young men with absolutely no specific training in how to handle a woman's body (other than the obvious lessons that they've picked up themselves after-hours). Now there's nothing wrong with young men. In fact, there are a lot of things awfully right about them. I can see a very good reason for regularly visiting a young ripped personal trainer at the gym every week. But don't expect him to provide all the answers to your weight-loss dreams. He would have to be a very special guy.

Most personal trainers will approach your weight-loss goals like this: tackle the bulge from the outside. Promote zero tolerance to fat and good old-fashioned sweat. Use weights and reps and presses and cardio and pump and spin — all designed to keep you alternating gym workouts with serial bursts of starvation for the rest of your natural life.

So. Here's some free advice.

Avoid personal trainers who promote pumping iron as the primary means of weight loss (unless they are very light weights used alongside other activities that raise your heart rate). Heavy weight training is good for people rehabilitating from injury or training for Ms Body Building Universe but for the rest of us . . . I'm not convinced. Call me stupid but I've never been able to work out why my life would be immeasurably better with a very strong *gluteus maximus* (bottom) muscle. Okay, so it's probably not a bad thing. Maybe having great gluts means you can wear G-strings more successfully? Or stand wearing them at all? If you know the answer to this, please email me. But if I had to choose a muscle to develop fully it wouldn't be my glut. It'd be the one inside my head: my brain.

But I digress. Again.

If you have the inclination — and the cash — to hire a personal weight-loss/activity trainer who can develop an individual plan to suit your own lifestyle, fine. Excellent, in fact. The one way in which personal trainers are guaranteed to work is that having someone at the gym waiting for you makes you go. Having a fitness/activity plan that is personally tailored to your needs and goals can help — but it isn't necessary. Most women go to the gym to lose weight — not to develop superb cardiovascular fitness. Therefore, we have basically the same needs: target the thighs, bum and stomach with a bit of toning around the arms. So all you really need in order to make some changes are a few guidelines.

Tip: The next time you reduce your food intake make sure you are physically active on a regular basis — or willing to introduce daily activity into your life. Because if all you do is cut your eating you will be training your already sluggish metabolism to operate on less food. And that equals disaster. You have probably been in that pattern over the years. I have met quite a few women who are a little overweight and actually eat very little. That's because they have brought their body, and metabolism, to a halt by not forcing it to move.

If you decrease what you eat NOW and increase what you do NOW, and keep doing it, then you WILL LOSE WEIGHT.

I lost 14kg over a whole year through a tough diet and an even tougher gym regime. I'm now a toned size 12 and I look as good as I've ever looked. I feel great. But I live in absolute terror that the weight is going to come back. I panic if I overeat or I miss the gym. Will I ever get to a point where I can relax, go to the gym for fun and not worry about my weight?
Georgia, 29

Dear Georgia,
I know your type. Not because I'm a psychologist. Just because I'm a woman. And every woman in the world wants to know the answer to this question. That is: how can you shove whatever you want in your mouth all day long and not gain a single kilo? Or, if you do, how you can strip the weight off again within a day? Sorry to disappoint, Georgia, you will never get to that point because no one ever does. Your body reflects your thoughts and your behaviour. You do, however, have a chance of relaxing (and skipping the odd gym class) if you can reset your mind to your great new look, then forget it, and go have some fun — outside the gym.

Tip: Try not to exercise on a totally empty stomach. But don't fill up just before you go as an excuse. Just eat naturally, the type and amount of food you think you need. And don't call it 'exercise' or a 'workout'. Don't be desperate about it. Just say I'm going for a walk or a swim or some time out. Just think about it like it's something you want to do. You don't have to behave like an Olympian. Just get out there. Grab an iPod, grab a friend, grab the kids if you don't have a choice. Just make it happen.

Going every day, even if it's just for a very short time, helps you to form good habits. But sometimes the weather, illness, injury or the family plays nasty tricks on you. When that happens, don't beat yourself up. Try to be active around the house. And as soon as you can, go again. Don't make it a chore. Start thinking of it as a fun thing to do. Some time out for yourself, a little pleasure and soon you won't want to miss and will start to look forward to it. And then you will have a new habit that will serve you well for life.

Food for thought

Physical education classes were boring but we should have listened.

Everything is activity. Even pegging out the washing. Even sex (but you have to try).

You have more chance of flying than becoming addicted to exercise.

Gyms don't make money from new customers.

Money won't help you lose weight. But that's no reason not to want it.

Activity that is fun for you is best. Actually, it's the only thing that works over time.

9 MY BUM WOULD LOOK BRILLIANT IF ... I LIKED MYSELF (EVEN WHEN TIME MESSES WITH MY BODY)

'You start out happy that you have no hips or boobs. All of a sudden you get them and it feels sloppy. Then just when you start liking them, they start drooping.' *Cindy Crawford, supermodel*

What do you think of yourself?

Good? Bad? Ugly? Self-esteem is the way we perceive our human worth. It's so important because of the impact it has on our thoughts and feelings and, so, on the quality of our lives. Good self-esteem gives us the confidence to take risks and go after the life we deserve; low self-esteem stirs feelings of guilt, shame and inadequacy that keep us trapped in a narrow and often miserable world. The broader concept of self-esteem is usually distinguished from self-confidence, which is more specific. So we may be confident about our ability to do certain things and to maintain certain relationships while struggling with more pervasive low self-worth.

In my experience people don't consistently think they are wonderful. Well, some do, but they are generally in jail or running the country, or they are people that wouldn't be much fun to hang out with. Most of us are much less convinced of our brilliance. Even on a good day, we are faking it. And we know that our self-view can change between the different spheres within which we work, play and live. So a lawyer with a history of messy relationships might rate herself highly professionally but be terribly insecure in the way she interacts with men. A woman who has been at home raising kids for years might rate her mothering ability but have no faith in her capacity to perform in a job — if she could muster up the confidence to go look for one.

What shapes our self-esteem

Self-esteem is shaped by personality traits, childhood and later experiences, feedback from other people and social beliefs built up around our appearance, achievements and relationships. The key traps people fall into that diminish self-esteem are comparing themselves with others, basing self-worth on tangible achievements and excessively seeking other people's approval. When women frequently say they 'don't fit' or have always felt on the fringe socially, it is often underpinned by a desperate need to be liked. Ironically (and sadly), this usually works against them: that is, when people sense your desperation they'll run in the opposite direction. And, if it's a man, he'll sprint.

Self-esteem is a tricky thing to measure because it can't be stuffed into categories of love or hate. It's not a neatly wrapped package and while most people from adolescence onwards have a self-esteem baseline, it can shift and wobble according to where we're at in our lives, who we're with (or not) and our circumstances. Some people believe that once your self-esteem level is set, you're stuck with it. But I'm in the camp that believes self-esteem can always be improved, that it's never too late to start feeling good about yourself.

Self-esteem and weight: what's the relationship?

A woman's self-esteem is frequently hooked to her physical appearance. Men, and forgive me for generalising but the trend is too marked to ignore, are more stuck on what they do. So it makes sense that women who are happy with their weight and looks feel good about themselves generally. Even better if they can maintain those feelings in the face of all that nature has to offer: pregnancy, midlife, menopause, hormonal problems — and all that goes with them.

Many women allow their weight and looks to dictate their opinion of themselves when I strongly believe it should be the other way around. Your weight should not be running the show. You should — and your weight should do as it's told. Feeling good about yourself is the key to losing weight and keeping it off. Women with low self-esteem can lose weight if they spend enough time away from the fridge and on the treadmill. But only women who are happy with themselves internally will be able to maintain that weight loss. (Read that sentence again, because it's really, really important.) Your weight depends on your happiness — NOT the other way around.

The way you behave in relation to food and activity is also dictated by your feelings about yourself. Why do you think bingeing is so common when women are stressed or miserable? When we are feeling bad about our lives or ourselves we don't care much (or even at all) what we shove into our mouths and its impact on our bodies.

What time does to women's bodies

Time really messes things up with women's bodies. Let's agree on that. As well as physical changes in our shape and weight distribution, we also have to confront the life stages linked to weight gain: adolescence, pregnancy, peri-menopause and menopause itself. It hardly seems fair: in terms of weight gain the only life stage men have to fear is the middle years. And the only raging hormones they have to live with are ours. Actually that's probably a reason to feel sorry for men. But only for a second. The exact point at which time asserts itself on our bodies is highly individual. All we know for sure is that at some point the distribution of weight begins to shift. Some of that shift is inevitable. What's not inevitable, though, is blowing out in uncomfortable and unhealthy proportions.

Handing your physical self over to time is a cop out. It's never okay to carry vast amounts of excess weight because it compromises your function and your health, not to mention your psychological wellbeing. You always have a say in how you look no matter how old you are — or feel.

The weight gain associated with midlife is distressing for women on two levels. Firstly, there's the panic over how to shift fatty deposits that have appeared in odd places and seem intent on staying despite your best efforts to shake them free. Secondly, women often struggle psychologically with the belief that their youth is over, that their physical attractiveness has packed up and left home for good.

JANE'S STORY

Physically, Jane was one of those women you envy. I wouldn't want to demean her long-standing struggle with anxiety but for me it was like looking at an older *Vogue* model complete with airbrushing. I felt seriously frumpy every time she came into my room. I found myself pulling out my most flattering outfits on Tuesdays when she had her regular appointment (I have insecurities too, remember). Anyway, Jane was a public relations consultant, newly separated and in her mid-40s, although she looked 10 years younger. She was about 185cm tall with legs that seemed to end about where my chin began. What bothered her was the newly rounded stomach and what she described as 'weird pouches' of fat on each side of her lower back that had developed over the past year.

'It's not fair,' she said. 'I haven't had kids, I'm not in the menopause, I go to the gym all the time and I'm still getting fat. What's going on?'

Jane knew the answer to that. She knew that time and nature were fully accountable for her weight gain. But when we unpacked her story, it wasn't her weight that bothered her most; it was her age and the physical toll that time was taking. Jane was terrified of getting older because every scrap of her self-worth was based on her looks: she'd been a beautiful kid who'd turned into a beautiful woman — and people had never stopped commenting on it. So although her anxiety was real, its source was fragile self-esteem built on a lifetime of looking good. In fact, Jane had lots of things going for her — she'd just never rated them as highly as her looks. Once she started to expand her own view of herself, there was no looking back and she made some big calls in terms of how she wanted to live. For the record, she's no longer in PR; she's off doing volunteer work somewhere like Borneo, having ditched the Zambesi for chain-store cargo pants and a faded T-shirt. And just to depress us all, she still looks fabulous.

Midlife weight gain and what it does to our heads

All women struggle with the physical impact of time to some degree. It's a rare woman who doesn't grimace when she looks in the mirror some mornings or long to look as young as she did in 10-year-old photos that she thought she looked hideous in at the time. But it seems to me that there are two groups of women who struggle most with their weight when they turn 30, have babies or hit any other age-related milestone:

1.   Those who got all the guys or gals. (Let's be politically correct.)
2.   Those who got none of the guys/gals.

1. Those who got all the guys/gals

These women were attractive teenagers who got plenty of attention and learnt how to use it. They grew up liking the way they looked. When the extra kilos start to appear in tandem with the wrinkles, they suffer. They pine for their lost youth. They think it's because they are losing their looks. But that's only a smoke screen; it's because they are losing their concept of what it means to be them, if they had ever fully developed it. They have to start again.

2. Those who got none of the guys/gals

These women struggled with their physical appearance all or most of their lives and grew up hating their looks. Those thoughts were reinforced by not getting much attention (at least not from the people they wanted it from). So their self-image was in tatters before they even fully matured. The first signs of age-related weight gain only compound that and they see their physical future as all downhill.

I'm not saying these are the only women who suffer from weight problems beyond the teenage years. We all do. Or nearly all of us. It's just that if you're a woman who falls into one of these groups it's useful to understand why you feel it so intensely. See, as I said before, it's not about the weight. It's about your concept of yourself. This is a really important topic so, be warned, we'll be going back there. But first we need to briefly consider some of the age-related reasons for weight gain — and what we can do about them.

Pregnancy

I've struggled with weight problems all my life so I'm terrified about what pregnancy will do to my body. I'm 10 weeks pregnant and already I'm eating more than I need because I've got a good excuse. And already I'm feeling guilty. I want a baby badly but the whole weight gain thing has pressed the panic button. What should I do? Guilty, 26

Dear Guilty,
Congratulations. Allow yourself a little joy, please. If you want a baby and you're in a good space to have one, then it's great news. As for the weight gain, pregnancy is a legitimate excuse. Repeat, legitimate. When you are pregnant you have to put on weight. Any other outcome is a disaster. There is one thing, though. When you are pregnant you have to eat well because you are eating for two. However, it's worth remembering that the other person you are eating for is the size of a golf ball, not the late Mama Cass. Don't use pregnancy as an excuse to eat double what you normally would, or it'll be a long, long road back to your current jean size.

'Guilty' probably represents a whole generation of women who deny themselves the joy of pregnancy (okay, it's not all joy for many of us) because of their weight-gain paranoia. Informal surveys suggest young women may delay having children because they don't want what they perceive as the weight issues that come with it. Who can blame them in a society that heralds hipbones over curves and suggests that while both thinness and motherhood are virtues, thinness is better. I've heard stories about how increasing numbers of young pregnant women are booking in for C-section deliveries two weeks earlier than their due date because it will cut down on the weight gain — and the stretch marks. It might also cut down on the ultimate health of the baby but — hey — why should that matter when you are thinking about how quickly you can get back into your jeans? Scary isn't it? Pregnancy equals weight gain. It's impossible to bear a healthy baby if you don't gain weight. Most women gain between 13 and 18kg each pregnancy, sometimes more, and obviously having multiple births raises the bar.

Post-pregnancy

Again, celebrity culture has much to answer for. One of the explosive media trends of the past 10 years is the celebrity post-baby body. Think about the number of stories in the women's magazines on how celebrities look after giving birth. One week we get the baby pictures; the very next we get the discussion on how quickly his/her famous mother can get her body back. Often the body beats the baby into print. Celebs who get the 'outstanding achievement' award are those who wear their pre-pregnancy jeans home from the hospital or delivery suite. Now there's an aspiration. But truly, the post-baby weight-loss race is on — and there is immense pressure to do it quicker than the next celeb. So be glad, be very glad, that the paparazzi haven't set up camp outside your house while you struggle with breastfeeding inside. Imagine the pressure. Women should be able to enjoy their pregnancy and get back to their pre-pregnancy form all in good time.

> I think I got really bad advice when I was pregnant. I got told not to worry about weight gain because it was a natural and normal part of the process, and that it would just come off later. Well, it hasn't. I had my second baby four years ago and none of the weight has shifted. Instead, I've ballooned to 20kg over my pre-pregnancy weight. Someone should have told me the truth.
> Eleanor, 41

Dear Eleanor,

First, some sympathy. Four years is a long time to be in the post-baby-weight zone because of the way it makes you feel about yourself. Having a baby takes a toll on your body. Actually that's understating it. It puts your body through the ringer; it pulls and stretches it in ways that you could have so done without. The older you are, the tougher it can be. Having kids can immerse you in a lifestyle that almost certainly won't be helping your weight. It's stressful trying to juggle everything and it's not just your body that is pulled and stretched in ways you didn't anticipate: it's your heart. So give yourself a break. Sure it's time to make some changes but go easy on yourself while you do it.

The 'middle' years

By the 'middle years', I mean the point at which gravity begins to exert its downward pull and the body decides to change its shape **without** our permission. It usually strikes between 30 and 45 years and bites hard psychologically because the redistribution of body weight, even when gradual, is evidence that a certain stage of our lives is over. The comforting thing is that it happens to us all, to some degree. Truly. If you have the body of a 19-year-old at 40 without sweating your life away in the gym then you are truly blessed. You might as well stop buying lotto tickets now because you've had your share of good fortune. If you were to win that as well you would have no friends. Ever. But I shouldn't be wasting words on this here, given that those extraordinarily rare women won't be reading this book. They'll be lying on a beach in a bikini.

Women's changing weight distribution in the middle years is a mean trick by nature and don't you wish she'd checked with us first. It goes like this: once we had an indentation between the breasts and the hips fondly referred to as our waist. Excess weight tended to sit on the hips, bum and thighs. But, in the middle years, extra padding begins to stick around the abdomen — and if it's already sticking there, you get more of it — so that the waist disappears. Strange little pouches of fat set up shop on the lower back and make us start shopping (discreetly at first, then what the heck) for bigger knickers and all-in-one body suits that hold all the bits in all the right places.

Simultaneously, gravity goes to work on the breasts and bum to give us the sag factor. I've never found proof as to whether this is due to the loss of elasticity of skin tissue or just an accumulation of bad habits; a little of both, probably. But suddenly it starts taking an awful lot of hours of activity to maintain any sort of shape at all. This is the point where many women give up and hit the bread bin, which, while understandable, is a very, very bad idea. You can control the gain — but not if you deliberately set about adding to it. A kilo here, a kilo there, is no big deal: it won't change the course of your life. But that same trend over five years isn't going to be a fun outcome at all. And if you don't exercise or at least keep physically active? Well, it'll probably just happen faster.

Peri-menopause, menopause and hormones

Women are lucky. Hold on, did I say lucky? Forgive me. Menopause is hardly a stroke of luck. What I mean is that menopause is a legitimate excuse for midlife weight gain, especially around the abdomen. And, let's face it, it sounds way better as an excuse than beer. We also have to acknowledge midlife hormones because they can make things tricky and spike our best efforts to lose and control weight. In fact, the clash of wayward hormones with midlife events such as relationship break-ups, loss of a parent and problems with children or career, can topple women into out-of-control eating and rapid weight gain.

Peri-menopause is to menopause what pregnancy is to motherhood. The warm up. The easy bit. (I'm not joking either. And at least, in theory, menopause ends.) But seriously, peri-menopause is the stage when you experience your first symptoms of menopause, such as night sweats, fluctuating hormones, hot flushes, fatigue, itchiness and rashes, insomnia and erratic periods. This stage is supposed to last for about 12 months before tipping us headlong into the real deal, which, as we all know, is more of the same — without the periods. Some would say it's nature's way of being kind but I think if nature was really in our corner it'd have let us lose the periods and skip all the other stuff too. It's all the proof I need that Mother Nature is a man.

That menopause, and the accompanying hormone replacement

medication, is linked with weight gain is well-documented. Even women who recovered their bodies entirely after pregnancies can't escape this one and the most slender of women will begin to thicken around the waist and to carry a 'menopot' out in front. On average that pot will add 2.2kg to our weight, which, looked at in context, shouldn't make much difference at all. But it does. Any weight gain hammers at our feelings about ourselves. Inversely, any woman who loses a little weight gets a boost to her self-esteem if not because of the associated praise then because she can go buy some new (smaller) clothes.

How do you rate yourself?

While midlife can toss up some specific weight challenges, being unhappy with your body/weight can take a psychological toll at any time because it can impact our:

- → Confidence
- → Sexiness and femininity
- → Communication style/skills
- → Social life
- → Pride
- → Respect
- → Relationships
- → Attitude
- → Self-image
- → View of our future

Have you ever noticed that when you are feeling great you eat less? Women in love often lose weight. That is not because they stop eating to please a partner. (Although I concede it might have something to do with having to peel your clothes off in front of someone for the first time.) Essentially, the reason women in love lose weight is because they feel good about themselves. They care. They have pride. Someone loves them. They stand straighter, their eyes sparkle — they stop focusing on food. People mistakenly believe it's because the new partner won't like what they see, but it's not.

Don't believe me? Have you ever noticed what happens when summer looms and you go to buy swimwear. In the changing room, every roll looks like an expansion pack of what you thought you had under your clothes so you instruct yourself: 'I must lose weight.' Yet you don't. You just let yourself feel bad. It should be a really good reason to do something about your weight — but it's not. The logic behind it is this: if you feel good about yourself most of the time, at least consistently, then you will manage your weight without even thinking about it. How's that for an idea? Imagine looking down, liking what you see, and having your body stay that way without giving it a thought. It's the same thing that happens when you break up with a partner or experience some grief in your life. It's not about the partner, per se. It's about what it does to your feelings of self-worth. For a while you don't care about yourself so you don't care how you treat yourself.

Some people react the other way. They can't eat, or don't, and immediately the weight falls off. But this spells equal trouble. The weight will be back, never fear. Because your weight is so connected to the way you feel about yourself, unless you can get some consistency around those thoughts you will never have stability around your weight.

Research shows that people who maintain consistent weight throughout their lifetime are happier, live longer, and lead fuller and more exciting lives. Yo-yo weight carriers are not. But perhaps that's the wrong way of looking at it. Because their lives are happy, their general levels of satisfaction are higher, so they are better placed to achieve physical consistency. I know what some of you are thinking: 'Ah, consistency is not my problem . . . I am consistently fat.' I see your point. And because I can't see you I can't see if you are being consistently honest.

STUFF TO DO: DO YOU FEEL GOOD (ENOUGH) ABOUT YOURSELF?

Let's think about your self-esteem. In other words, what you think of yourself, your feelings of self-value or -worth. Draw a line on the scale where you think you fit.

1   10

Loathe myself   *Love myself*

[All 10s please close the book now. You can't stay here. You will just depress the rest of us.]

Now ask these questions:

Are you satisfied with your rating?

What would it take to get to 10?

Think carefully. Would weight loss on its own do the trick? Or are there other areas of your life that could do with a boost? Your work or career? Your relationships?

Does weight loss alone hold the key to changing your life?

If you can't get past weight loss, what else would make your life better? Try to break down your life into areas. The more specific you can be, the better.

Building up your self-esteem

If you have high self-esteem, skip this section. Stick with me if yours is towards the lower end of the scale, or you think it could do with a lift.

Your self-esteem or sense of self-worth can be increased. But I've never bought into that whole positive affirmation thing, especially where a woman's body is concerned, because our negative beliefs about our bodies are so entrenched. Sticking little love notes to yourself on the fridge or standing in front of a mirror repeatedly saying 'I love you, I love you, I love you' is futile. I read somewhere that you should do this naked. I have no idea whose idea this was but it's not a good one. It won't work. It's sadistic. It may even make you feel worse because you will think you are lying to yourself. The people you live with will think you're weird if they see the notes or come in while you're standing there doing it. And it's kind of creepy too. If you don't believe me, try it. You'll find it's a dodgy way to spend your time.

STUFF TO DO: WHY YOU ARE WORTHY

Your self-esteem is largely based on how you gauge your own achievements and on your acceptance and appreciation for the things you have in your life. It's less about the things you have done and more about you **being aware of and appreciating** the things you have done: on finding and acknowledging evidence for your achievements. I'm not just talking about work: pinning your self-worth to your career or job is narrow, not to mention dangerous for your psychological health.

1. Your achievements

So what have you done in your life? Don't hit me with 'I've done nothing' because unless you've been in bed since birth then you have done something. It's likely, however, that from this point on you want to be — and should be — doing more with your life. That's a good thing. You can build up your sense of achievement by taking action, one task at a time, one day at a time.

Now, working quickly, name six things you have done in your life. Don't worry if these things seem insignificant to you; just note the first six things that pop into your head. Try to think broadly across all areas of your life: family, friends, interests, work, health, money, education, travel and the like. If you're struggling, try to recall times in which you felt good and think about what you were doing at the time. Write them down; this particular exercise works better if you do.

1. _____

2. _____

3. _____

4 _____

5. _____

6. _____

2. Self-appreciation

Now here's the second part. Again, working quickly, write down six things that you like about yourself as a person. Not anything to do with your job, career, looks, achievements or possessions. Just human qualities — things that would draw you to other people if they demonstrated them.

1. _____

2. _____

_____

3. _____

_____

4. _____

_____

5. _____

_____

6. _____

_____

I'm hoping that was easy for you. It should have been because everyone has done something with their life — and everyone has some worthwhile human qualities. The hard part sometimes, especially when we are being self-critical, is being aware of and appreciating the good in ourselves. But in every woman — in every person — there's always lots to love. It just takes some people a while to find or acknowledge this. Remember, acknowledging yourself and your achievements is crucial in boosting your self-worth and you have to do that if your weight is ever going to settle, and stay, at a level you are happy with.

Chances are, if you are reading this book, then you are not thrilled with who you are. Or at least what you look like. But often it goes further than that: frequently the reason women put on or carry excess weight is that they don't rate themselves highly enough to do something about it. They don't think they are worth it. Which is about the saddest thing that I hear, because you are SO worth it. Note: It's not unusual to struggle with these exercises. If you have found them tough, don't despair. The next section will help you.

STUFF TO DO: WHO ARE YOU?

Women who want to lose weight often host a harsh internal critic, a voice that gets in their ear day after day just to remind them of all their perceived weaknesses and defects. The best way to silence this critic is to focus on our strengths and interests.

So who are you? Remember I asked that question back near the beginning of the book. Now it's time to answer it. I know it seems like a big question — but that's no reason to dodge it. Most people do. Some avoid it because they don't want to know the answer, but most just don't think to ask the question. That's not smart, though, because knowing yourself is the first step in leading a full and satisfying life. How else can you make the necessary changes?

So how do you figure it out? The first step is to think about what you enjoy doing and what you are good at. These help set down a baseline for things you look to increase in your life. Try to think beyond what you are doing right now. Think about what you've done in the past and what you would like to do in the future. If you are thinking about work you have done, try to be specific about what areas/tasks you most enjoyed and in which you demonstrated the most skill.

What do you love to do?

What are you good at?

Put these two headings at the top of the page. Now write yourself two lists. If you like, you can do it in two overlapping circles like the diagram over the page. Don't be too academic about it. Just put the brain in free fall and fill the page.

Finished? Sometimes it pays to leave it a few days and add some more. If you're struggling, ask friends and family members to help. Often they see your talents and interests more clearly than you do, especially at times when you're feeling a little down.

Now ask . . .

Which things have you written on **both** lists or in **both** circles? These are a clue to what you should be doing more of. Pick one of them. What could you do today to introduce more of this thing into your life? The smallest step counts, such as looking on the internet or making a phone call. The only rule is that you have to do it today. Or tomorrow if you're in bed reading this. But leave it any longer and you're slipping into the procrastination zone, which won't make you feel good about anything, including your body.

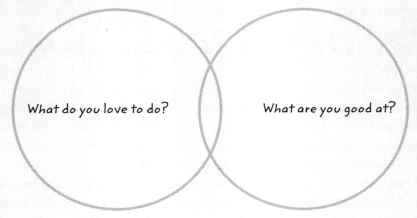

Food for thought

Sooner or later nature and gravity will turn against you and your weight.

But there's a limit — and you have to impose it.

Some people think they are wonderful. These people are smart.

Some people think they are wonderful and tell you so. These people are boring.

Your happiness should dictate your weight — not the other way around.

Feeling good about yourself is the most important thing of all. Seriously.

10 MY BUM WOULD LOOK BRILLIANT IF . . . MY FAMILY AND FRIENDS WOULD HELP ME

'I was married for 30 years. Isn't that enough? I've had my share of dirty underwear on the floor.' *Martha Stewart, domestic goddess*

People are our greatest joy. They also present us with our biggest challenges. When our relationships go right they give us a reason to be here, to feel wanted and loved and part of something. When they go wrong they leave us sad, shaken, angry and often desolate. And yet we crave them. Loneliness in its various forms underpins so much depression and sadness. Love, feeling special and wanted, finding our place, is essential to our happiness. But the quest for love often takes us in all the wrong directions, leaves us with bruises and scars, and stretches us thin to transparency. It makes us land in places that are not soft after all. Just because love is the greatest thing, doesn't mean it's the easiest.

Our relationships affect our health, wellbeing and — of course — our weight. And I'm not just talking about intimate relationships: I'm also talking about family, friends, work colleagues and anyone else who occupies our inner sphere. These people influence our behavioural choices, including those we make around food and eating. So when we are with some people we eat too much of the wrong stuff, when we are with others we eat the right food in healthy proportions. What does all this mean? Nothing, really — even though many weight-loss experts suggest you should be spending more time with people who make all the right food choices. That's fine in theory, but who is so committed to weight loss that they move in with another family or dump their friends to hang out with skinny people? Hopefully no one reading this book is that fickle. Besides, who wants to choose their social circle based on how and what they eat? What boring criteria. The important thing is to notice how the people in your life 'use' food. And then, if you don't like what you see, make a deal with yourself to do things differently.

I'm about 15kg overweight. My partner Pete is about the same. But while I spend every waking minute thinking about what I'm eating — or shouldn't be — he spends no time at all. He doesn't care about what he eats and what he weighs. And he tells me I shouldn't care either. He says he loves me big or small or any old how.
Pete's gal, 47

Dear Pete's gal (please use your own name next time. I want you to be your own person not some guy's man bag),
I would say lucky you, but I don't know Pete. Maybe you're not so lucky? I do know this though: our men are nowhere near as hung up about our weight as we are. If they love us, they love us. A few kilos makes no difference to them. If a man is picking at you about your weight, it may reflect dissatisfaction with his own life or his own insecurities. It's possible that an overweight man might feel more comfortable with a woman in his own weight league. But he might not either. Give Pete the benefit of that doubt. Maybe he just loves you. Why wouldn't he? Get yourself feeling fabulous in all areas of your life and if you're both still happy then I love that. It puts you way ahead of pretty much everyone else.

They love me. So why won't they help me?

One of the toughest things about losing weight is trying to elicit support from our favourite people. But while it's a nice idea, it's just not realistic to expect everyone around us to jump on board with our plans. Even people who love us will sometimes undermine our best efforts — often just because they're busy dealing with their own lives. But some people will want you to stay as you are so they don't feel guilty (or you don't run off with someone else); some are too lazy to help you; and some people just want someone (you) to join them in eating large amounts of food because it's more fun than doing it alone. A few will actively sabotage your best intentions. Which is a total pain. But — remember — whether they succeed or not is up to you.

So what should you do?

Wanting to detour or derail those who interfere with your efforts to lose weight is not enough. You need to have a specific plan in mind for how to deal with them. The best way is to use a four-step approach. Answer the following questions:

1. **Who** is ruining my weight-loss efforts?
2. **How** are they doing it?
3. **Why** are they doing it?
4. **My response**: what can I do to produce a different outcome?

The key is to consider **why** these people are sabotaging your efforts? Consider each of them separately. Is their sabotage intentional or not? Is it a nurturing act or a mean-minded one? Are they acting on their own fears and insecurities? Are they jealous? Are they worried that a change in how you look will have an impact on them?

Once you have figured out the reason they are putting up a barrier, it's much easier to figure out a counter-response. So if a friend keeps inviting you for coffee because she's lonely you can suggest doing something more active instead. And if a partner thinks a new, slim you may run off into the arms of a new lover you can come up with a way to alleviate that fear (unless that is exactly what you are planning and, if so, I'm not helping you with an excuse. Good luck, though.)

Fact: People are fearful about what change means for **their** lives. **Not yours**. So try to see your efforts to lose weight through their eyes. It will help you work out the best way to deal with their resistance.

Further fact: Some people will never want you to change and will do everything they can to keep you the same. You have to decide how much you want to change **and** whether these people are worth staying the same for.

STUFF TO DO: **WHO'S IN YOUR LIFE?**

In the left-hand circle below write the names of the six people you spend the most time with (in no particular order and don't include children). Don't make it all about family. It's okay to lump family members together; the idea is to get a picture of who you mostly hang out with.

In the other circle, write the names of the people you most enjoy spending time with. Who inspires you? Who are the people who make you feel good about yourself? Or about your life?

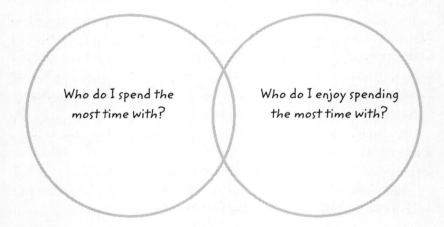

Who do I spend the most time with?

Who do I enjoy spending the most time with?

What does this mean?
Check which names appear in both circles. Frequently there is not much crossover. Generally, we spend the most time with those who we work and live with. Often it is very hard to get time with your friends: people with whom you can fully relax and who uplift you.

Now, next to the names of your friends, write down the quality that makes you most want to be with them. For example: someone to go out on the town with, help with the kids, walking/gym buddy, good listener, professional advice, 'gets me', a good laugh.

Often we get different things from different people and that's a good thing. But the key thing to remember is that you and the way you are is most influenced by the six or so people with whom you spend the most time. So if your world's not feeling great right now, consider the ratio of who's bringing what to your life: it might need a tweak. And if there's no one in your life that you have fun with then it needs a major overhaul.

Now think about the people in your life in terms of your weight. If you hang out with a lot of very big people then you are likely to adopt the same thinking and behaviour around food that they have. Or at least maintain the habits that are causing your problems. As I said before, I'm not saying you have to find yourself a bunch of skinny friends (that might trigger some other self-esteem issues) but it may be time to consider the ways in which the company you keep impacts on your health.

A good way to move forward is to take a look at the lifestyle of someone whom you consider has it all together — and work out how you could achieve that. How does that person eat? What is their relationship with food? Observe them. Ask them. Most people won't mind. More importantly look not just at how they are around food, look at how they are with life. And, if you like what you see, then try to spend a little more time with them. Not in a stalking way though, or they'll be off running.

Does the perfect woman exist?

Human perfection is an elusive state. It's also a really dumb goal because when you don't achieve it (and you won't) you will feel even worse about yourself than you do now. So what's perfection in a woman? Come on, think about it. How many women do you know who meet all of these six criteria:

1.   Slim (without eating like a sparrow).
2.   Rich (enough to be a haute couture clothes horse, have a gorgeous home and regular Caribbean holidays).
3.   Healthy (without spending more on gym memberships than she does on shoes).
4.   Fun (gets a joke and isn't afraid to tell one).
5.   Successful at work.
6.   Enjoys great relationships with **all** the people in her life?

How many did you come up with? I can only think of one: her name was Wonder Woman, the greatest female superhero of all time. And you have to say that flying round all day in a scant bikini (without body image insecurity) equals a pretty easy life. She didn't have to deal with a tired relationship, money worries and sick kids. And I bet she didn't have to clean the house.

The truth is that hardly anyone scores six out of six. Most of us are flawed. That's what makes us fun. I really would hate to be perfect. (Hmm. Okay, I lie. You saw right through that one, didn't you?) But think about it: those who appear seriously happy are usually drunk. The rich are often fat; the slim are often living on their nerves and insecurities. Show me the woman who has it all and I'll show you an alien being. She doesn't exist, except in our minds. And someone planted her there just to make it hard for us. To make us think the impossible dream was possible after all. And we bought it. Silly old us.

The people in your life
Partners

Partners — or the lack of them — are key players in our beliefs about our bodies and our efforts to lose weight. Many women blame their partners for maintaining their weight problems and undermining their attempts to change. Single women often think their weight is a barrier to them finding Mr Right. Which it is if Mr Right is actually Mr Superficial (and therefore Mr Wrong in disguise). Let's face it — when it comes to our weight, male partners haven't got a chance. Women are genius at twisting anything a man says, or does, to help us feel bad about ourselves. Don't believe me? Then consider where your partner or previous partners fit into this list:

→ If he's happy with your weight, then he's not being supportive of your efforts to lose it.
→ If he's not happy with your weight, then he's not loving you for who you are.
→ If he fails to notice a 3kg drop in your weight then he's not appreciating the effort you've put in.
→ If he does notice that 3kg reduction then that just proves how conscious he is of your weight. Or perhaps he's gay. Gay men get all this stuff.
→ And if he manages to negotiate the minefield that is all this, then he's wasted as a man. He needs to be a woman. Of course the right response to any question asked of a man, or even any situation, is 'Your bum looks brilliant in everything, darling,' but astonishingly very few guys figure this out.

Note: If you have a female partner then in theory the whole weight-loss thing should be easier because she should understand. But it's not. Two female minds are harder to navigate than one and even more scary if you are both trying to lose weight.

My partner tells me I'm too fat. It's true that I'm fatter than him but he's built like a pretzel. What should I do?
Fatter than my guy, 43

Dear Person,
I refuse to use your pseudonym because it's not kind and you're comparing yourself to someone else. Even worse, you're comparing yourself to a guy! How does that work? Okay, I can't see you so he might have a point. What are you too fat for? Too fat is when you can't comfortably live the life you were designed to live. Do you huff and puff with physical effort? Can you play touch with your workmates or run around the park with your kids or dog? Do you have plenty of energy for all the things you'd like to do? If you think

you are amazing, then you are amazing. But I suspect that because you are telling me this you are bothered by your weight. It might be time to do something about it. But do it for you and because you want to have a better life. Not because your pretzel-thin bloke says so. By the way, is he too skinny for you? If he is, it might be time to tell him.

Your family

If we want to keep the complexity out of this — and I always do — there are two family compositions that affect your weight and body image:

→   Your family of origin, which is the one you were born into and/ or raised in.
→   The family you are immersed in right now, that you have either created, been drawn into or just sort of landed among, including flatting situations.

Both of these have all sorts of variations in form, ranging from adopted to blended to step to extended to convenient and so on. And both of these have all sorts of variations in satisfaction and harmony levels from loving to laid-back to cruisey to conflict-ridden to downright bloody awful.

The only reason we need to consider families here is in terms of their impact on your weight, body image and attitude to food and exercise. We've already discussed the influence of your family of origin: that is, your biology, your early food environment and the development of your body image. If you are still living with these people then these things are still a consideration for you. It might just be that it's time to move out. But that's over to you. I'm not in the business of breaking up families — or forcing you to set up your bed on a park bench just because you and the family don't have compatible ideas about food.

Because I've written this book for women aged between 25 and 50 years approximately (if you don't quite make the cut you're still welcome), I'm thinking that most of you have left the folks behind and moved on. So the question you need to ask is: are the people you live with helping you (or at least not undermining you) in your efforts to lose and maintain weight?

- → If the answer is 'yes' then that's good. Make yourself at home because this is working for you.
- → If the answer is 'no' then you have three choices: move out (probably tempting but perhaps not practical), force them to eat like you want to (will probably cause a fight) or do your own thing (easily the best alternative, although it has challenges).

Many women say their best efforts to lose weight get thwarted by family food demands and needs. It makes sense, doesn't it? You only want to cook one evening meal; you haven't got enough money to buy large quantities (for the whole family) of the healthier food you'd like to eat; you don't want to fill the fridge with tasty healthy food for yourself because the insects (people other than you who inhabit your house) will scoff it (probably while you're asleep). I know, I know, it's difficult. The only workable solution is to cook reasonably simple good food for the family and just eat less of it yourself. Even with the best intentions, anything else gets too hard after a while and you'll give up.

I'm worried. No, I'm panicking. I weigh 20kg more than I did two years ago. I don't know where the weight is coming from, but it just keeps coming. If it's middle-age spread then I've got it big time. But why? I've got a good life, although I get pretty wound up over my husband and three kids. We've moved town. I wish we had more money. And I don't know what to do next. Do you think that's got something to do with it?
Confused, 41

Dear Confused,
Have you ever thought of studying psychology? You don't need me. You understand yourself perfectly. It's not about your weight. It's my guess you've been so busy slaving after your family for years you've lost sight of yourself. You are so not alone in this. I call it the 'Now What?' syndrome. It's endemic. It mostly strikes women whose children have all gone off to school and they suddenly realise they have no plan for themselves for the next 40 years. Forget your weight (but please don't eat for the starving inhabitants of Africa).

Find something meaningful to do (and get help with this bit if you need to), something for yourself, that you enjoy. Then start doing it. Do lots of it if you can. The weight will take care of itself.

Six months later *Confused* wrote back . . .

I got it. I got it. I've been an office administrator most of my working life. I was good at it but it was just a job and I didn't want to go back there after we moved. So I decided to follow up on my favourite hobby. Now I'm working at my local garden centre and I've done a couple of small landscaping jobs for friends — and been paid for it! At nights I read garden and landscaping books and I'm thinking of doing some more study. I get to spend all day in my gumboots. I feel more energetic and healthy — and I've even lost a bit of weight. I still run around crazily after my family but it doesn't matter so much now that I've got something of my own.

A note for mothers:

Whether you are with your kids 24/7 or have another job as well, being a mother is demanding and relentless — and that's on a good day when no one is throwing food, melting down or beating up on a brother or sister. That, sadly, is often the fun part. The tough bit is that you are left with no time for yourself, and that includes eating well, exercising and non-child-related FUN. A few women can build their lives wholly around their children. Many businesses have been born out of all that crawl time on the floor — and that's great. For them. Most of us need to work outside the home — both to earn money and to have another outlet for our energies — if we are going to have any hope of being decent mothers. We need something else meaningful to do even if it's not right at the point when we are up to our necks in mushy food (which for some puzzling reason is called solids). Most of us need to have a stake in the future so that on those really, really boring days when the kids lose it with tantrums and throw up on our best black clothes we have something else to think about; we can at least send our mind out for a coffee break.

Many women are waiting . . . waiting . . . until the kids get a lot older (go to school, secondary school, leave home) to do something for themselves. But here's a question: when the kids leave home do you still want to be doing a job/activity that you fitted around their pre-school activities? While you might be a little constrained right now, it's worth thinking about how you want your life to be in five or 10 years' time. Possibly the best thing you can do for your kids as they grow up is to start doing something meaningful for yourself, even if it's on the smallest scale. So that by the time they leave home (and hopefully they do), you will be flying. In the meantime you will enjoy your life more. You will be more fulfilled and interesting — and it will stop you thinking about food. And you will have something else to think about when your teenagers drive you crazy. Because they will.

Your friends

Your friends are your friends; if they are good ones they will care what you weigh because it bothers **you**, not because it bothers them. They will have your best intentions at heart even if they don't strip the skin off the chicken before they cook it for you. If they are the other type, what are you thinking? We should be accommodating with people but not suckers for them. The rule is this: if people generally bring good things to your life, then keep them. If not, then maybe it's time to put in a little distance?

A lot of people claim they would like to have new or more friends but a) don't have the time/energy to put into building these relationships or b) don't like doing 'small talk'. I'm not listening to the 'small talk' excuse: if you are bored in a conversation then maybe you are being boring? You just might need to ask better questions. Lack of time and energy for new friendships, however, is a legitimate excuse because relationships need both of those things. But don't be in too much of a rush: forcing friendship doesn't generally bring the desired results. Sometimes things just evolve over time, and friendships that take months or years to develop are often the best of all. This I will concede though: some people just might not be good friendship material for you. Here's a trick you can use in social situations — I made it up after a few years of experimentation and a (very popular) friend of mine swears by it. When you meet someone new ask them five questions about themselves. Show genuine interest in the person, don't fire the questions at him/her machine-gun style. If, after five questions, the person has asked you nothing about yourself in return then it's a signal to move on. This person probably has some fine qualities. But the reality is that they are probably not going to invest much time in finding out what yours are.

The people you work with

Does it really matter what your colleagues or workmates think of your weight and what you eat? Only if they are your friends or you are having an affair with one of them. If they are your friends, see the above section. And even if you are having a dangerous liaison, I'd lay money down that this person does not pack your lunch every day. Remember you don't have to eat cakes and pies every time someone at work shouts morning tea. **You** are in charge of what you eat. Not a bunch of people who are fine at work but who often seem a little weird, and oddly dressed, when you see them in real life. If, of course, you work in one of those ridiculously fun social places where food is part of the culture, people graze constantly, and you can't control yourself in the staff kitchen (with the food), it might be time to dust off the CV and prepare your farewell speech.

When people matter too much

Sometimes we get frustrated with people because we are looking to them to save, heal or improve our lives. Often we don't even realise it. This often underpins some women's quest for a long-term partner. The truth is that while a partner might make you feel better temporarily (and may ultimately make you feel worse), he or she won't guarantee you everlasting happiness. In fact, the more you lean on a relationship to improve your life the more likely you are to destroy it. I am always astonished how many women think a man is the answer to all their problems. Why would they ever think that? Men are great but if you've ever lived with one you will know that they are often the beginning of your problems — not the end of them. Apart from the biological drive to reproduce, and sex if he is really good at it, I can't identify a good enough reason for obsessing over a man. There are other ways to do both of those activities. Please don't think I am anti-men because I am actually very pro-men. Men are interesting, think and act differently, and are often very cute — and that's the appeal. They should not have to be our saviours. Just as we should not have to be theirs. The knight in shining armour riding in on a white stallion is only cool if you believe in fairytales. And if you have room in your house for a horse.

Sorry, but the job of being fabulous is yours. It can't be delegated. Make yourself amazing and good people, men and women, will start to trail after you.

The strange twenty-first century phenomenon of work–life balance

Everyone goes on about work-life balance as the ultimate twenty-first century goal. I find it a little strange: I don't know about you but I'm not aiming to have someone say 'She achieved really good work-life balance' about me at my funeral. I would rather have some of my good qualities mentioned and hope people forget about all the others. Work-life balance or life balance, as some people prefer, are just fresh spins on the concept of living well, which has been around since the beginning of time, or at least since the ancient Greek philosophers worked out there was more to life than tossing a discus and scoffing down figs. What it comes down to is that all any person has is the interval between now and when it's over — so our only obligation is to use that time as well as we can. It is, and has always been, in our best interest to create full and interesting lives. But it's even more important to live our lives according to our own beliefs and values. If you like to work there is no reason why you shouldn't do an awful lot of it as long as all other spheres of your life aren't falling apart and your favourite people aren't yelling at you. The best way to assess it is to imagine that your life will be over by the end of the week. Would you be able to rest easily at your own funeral or would you be ashamed of what you haven't done and/or guilt-stricken about people you should have spent time with? If you feel a hint of guilt (which of course you will if you are a woman) then it may be time to make some changes. The adjustments you need to make are often more about shifting your priorities than getting a perfectly weighted work-life balance.

Some facts to make the task easier:

→ If you like your job, you will work a lot. But if you're smart you will sometimes stop working and go talk to your partner/kids/family/friends/other people because if you don't you will be very boring (and lonely).

→ If you like certain people you will spend a lot of time with them. But if you're smart you will sometimes leave them alone and go earn some money, study or do other things because if you don't you will be very boring (and shallow . . . and possibly broke).

→ If you like doing leisure/pleasure activities, you will do a lot of them. But if you're smart you will do more with yourself than just these activities because if you don't you will be very boring (and bored). Truly. The fun quickly goes out of leisure activities when you've got nothing else going on — although I concede that it's pretty nice for a while.

You can tell I have a thing about being bored and boring, and I think everyone should. If you don't get involved with a variety of people, interests and activities you won't have much to talk or think about and, therefore, you will find it hard to make and maintain relationships. Imagine going out for a drink with Florence Nightingale or Marie Curie? Hearing about their deeds might be uplifting but if you're not into hospitals or radium it might get a little dull after a while. Okay probably not, but the point is that we should strive not for work-life balance but to make ourselves fuller, more interesting people. We may or may not have succeeded when our time is up, but at least we'll have tried a few things along the way.

How to be a more interesting person (or how to set non-weight-related goals so you can get on with living)

Generally, when women are unhappy with their bodies or want to lose weight, the first thing they do is set a weight-related goal. Actually, it's the only thing. That is not smart behaviour because it pins success or achievement to losing weight. Everything else you do loses significance. It also makes losing weight the BIGGEST thing in your life — and we've already discussed at length the problem with that. So you need to set goals **not** related to your weight. And, to do that, you need to think more generally about your life, your satisfaction with it and where you believe it is heading. How do you want your life to turn out? What kind of person do you want to be? Do you have a clear, or even vague, view of your future?

More than 90 per cent of the population can't answer these questions. Not because they're incapable, just because they've never tried. Most people are content to fall out of bed each day, put one foot in front of the other and end up 'somewhere or other'. Actually, they're not all content. If only. Many are dissatisfied, unhappy and desperate. That's because they have no direction and it makes their existence seem dull and futile. Many people plan their finances, holidays, kids' activities, and even their working days with meticulous attention. But their lives? The biggest and longest event they'll ever participate in and they just let it roll out day-by-day for 75-plus years without a plan. It scares me because the results of all this unhappiness and vagueness end up on couches like mine.

So you need a plan. Plans are based on achievable steps, otherwise known as goals. Goal setting is a very old concept. Some people carry their plans in their heads. That's fine. Others have a goal-setting phobia and, if that's you, you can skip this section. But the easiest way to reboot your life or to boost it up in certain areas is to set some goals. If you are depressed, it is crucial. There are many, many books, websites, articles — and experts — that can help in this area. So if you are interested, you should explore it further. In the meantime I just want you to think about how satisfying your life is to **you** right now and which areas of it could do with a tweak. This is not about finding your 'passion' or 'true calling', which I'll touch on in the final chapter. All you need are some interesting things to do, some interesting people to do them with, a picture of how you'd like your life to be — and a plan for getting there.

Framing your future

Step 1: The big picture

The first step is to think about the kind of person you are. If you need help return to the chart you filled out in chapter 9. What are you good at? What do you love doing? Allow yourself to think beyond your life as it is right now. Think back to when you were a child. Think forward to what you'd like to be doing in 10 years. Think about your work, your hobbies, your relationships, your family and home, your finances, interests, spiritual values. Think big because in a minute I'll ask you to think small.

Step 2: In 10 years

Form a picture of where you would like to be in all aspects of your life in 10 years. What kind of person would you like to be? What would you like to be doing? You can do this with words but it's often more powerful to build a visual picture on an A4 sheet (or larger). I've seen women come up with some amazing things: the more you can come up with the more excited you will feel about your short- and long-term future.

Step 3: The smaller picture

Set yourself some tasks under the headings below. Think about every area of your life — work, study, family, friends, social, hobbies, recreation/leisure, health, sport, finances, home, travel, spiritual, and so on — except your body and weight.

Tip: Be as specific as you can and write down as many things as you can. This is a work in progress so you don't have to do it all in one hit (in fact, many people find this difficult). Come back to it.

My goals for:

The next month

_____

_____

_____

The next six months

The next year

The next three years

The next five years

182 My bum would look brilliant if . . .

Step 4: Taking action

'The journey of a thousand miles begins with one step.'
Lao Tzu, philosopher

Setting goals without taking action is obviously no use at all. The trick is to think small. Do small things one at a time. Then do more of them. If you think about the big picture all the time it will seem too hard and you'll end up procrastinating and doing nothing. So if you are an artist, you are thinking one brush stroke, one hour, one painting at a time. If you are an athlete, it's one skill, one training session, one event at a time. I always think everyone should run one marathon in their lifetime — no, forget that, I'd hate it. But marathon running offers the ultimate proof that one step at a time brings results. Or every little thing you do is progress.

The key to success is **daily action**. Make sure you do one thing each day to move yourself towards your goals, feel the sense of achievement at having done something, and then relax.

Food for thought

Relationships are the source of our greatest joy. They can also be a pain in the, er, bum.

A man can be the beginning of your problems — not the end of them.

If all your friends are skinny you need to make more (or bigger) friends.

If you fill your fridge with healthy food then the other people in your house will eat it.

Most people don't know where they're going. But they're hell bent on getting there.

Work-life balance is a dull new spin on the importance of living fully.

Set goals not related to your weight. Make them small. Tiny, even. Then you'll do them.

11 MY BUM WOULD LOOK BRILLIANT IF ... I COULD KEEP WEIGHT OFF AFTER LOSING IT

'I never do any television without chocolate. That's my motto and I live by it. Quite often I write the scripts and I make sure there are chocolate scenes. Actually I'm a bit of a chocolate tart and will eat anything. It's amazing I'm so slim.' *Dawn French, comedian and actor*

It is said there are two certainties in life: death and taxes. A third is that we will make mistakes. I don't want to talk about taxes. Nor dying because this book is about living — and it's important that while we are on the vertical side of the line we do it as well as we can. But we need to talk about mistakes because we have to make them in order to live fully. I'm far from perfect so I don't expect you to be. You are allowed to be stupid and/or mess up for at least five minutes every day. Just try not to go over that limit. Well not every day, anyway.

Achieving lasting weight loss isn't a robotic march to the Kingdom of the Brilliant Bum. I didn't promise that at the start of this book and if anyone does you should run away from them faster than you would from a used-car salesman with gold teeth. If you are trying to lose weight you **will** screw up. Sometimes you will eat the wrong food. Sometimes you will eat too much of it. Sometimes you will eat too fast or on the run. Not because you are flawed, or even because you are a woman. Because you are human. But managing your weight is not like managing a class-A drug addiction. Sneaking one piece of cake does not have the potential to ruin your life. It will only do that if you think so obsessively about that cake — before and after you have eaten it — that you feel compelled to hunt down another slice. Then another. And so on.

I'd been overweight since my teens. I left home at 18 to go to university, began drinking beer and eating stodgy food and started to put on weight. I never lost it; I just got bigger. Over the years I've tried heaps of diets with various (not much) amounts of success. So two years ago I got serious, joined a weight-loss group and put in a huge effort. I lost the most weight of anyone in a year — not just in our group but in the whole region. My prize was a new wardrobe and I got featured in a women's magazine. Everyone was congratulating me and I felt on top of the world. But when all that hype died down I went back to normal life and I've started to gain weight again. Not much yet, but I wake up every morning with a feeling of dread. It's like walking on eggshells. I'm panicking. I know the statistics. I'm going to be even bigger than before, aren't I?
Panic Artist, 37

Dear Panic Artist (also known as crystal-ball gazer),
Yes, unless you break the cycle, you're going to be bigger than before. I know this only because you're telling me you know it. You are visualising yourself at your all-new enormous weight — and you are doing it while you are still slim! That's sad. Please, allow yourself to enjoy the results of all your hard work. That's why I have a problem with most weight-loss programmes — they only focus on reducing your size, they conveniently forget about helping you to stay there or on helping you create a more meaningful life. Once you've lost weight you have to programme your mind to handle your new look. You have to shift from weight loss to weight maintenance mode. And you absolutely have to do something meaningful with your life other than think about your weight. So, come on, be the best person in your group at keeping the weight off — it'll really make you happy.

If you've ever tried to lose weight (and you're still trying) you've made mistakes. I refuse to call them failures because if you're still trying to lose weight you're still in the game. And, besides, I'm one of those annoying people who believes failure is simply an opportunity to more intelligently (or creatively) begin again. If you don't fail sometimes then are you actually doing anything? Or are you just at home hiding under your bed? For now, let's just think of your past mistakes as difficulties.

So, for the record, these are the two most commonly reported difficulties in weight loss:

1. Never getting properly started (or a 'stop-start' pattern of dieting/exercise).
2. Regaining weight once you've lost it.

1. Never getting properly started

Instant gratification is a catch-cry of modern existence. When we decide we want something, we want it NOW and we want it FAST. We don't want to pay our dues, even though we know we should, because **we don't have time**. We are all in such a rush. Check out how many people jab at the door-close buttons in elevators just to gain a few seconds in their day. So it is often the slowness of weight loss (in combination with our unrealistic goals) that causes us to stumble when we've been doing really well. It's interesting psychologically because even though we gain weight over months/years, we expect to lose it over days/weeks. And when we don't, we're put off, we start thinking it's all too hard. All the (sensible) diet gurus say the same thing: cut down food slowly and sensibly and you are on your way.

In theory I don't have a problem with that because that's what you have to do. Except that this approach doesn't fully take into account one of the fundamentals of the human psyche. That is, if we are going to give up something we love we want to get some payback. Dieting demands that we give up our culinary pleasures slowly, one day at a time and **keep doing it for life**. That's where it gets you — right there — the words 'for life' ring in your ear like a prison sentence. Further, the rewards or the signs of change are so incremental, so slow, that they can barely be noticed. So you starve yourself for two weeks, hop on the scales and you've lost 1.5kg. Then you weigh yourself the next day and you have put it back on. That measly 1.5kg that you strived so hard to lose has found its way back — and it's done it while you slept. How disheartening. No wonder we give up.

2. Regaining weight once you've lost it

We've all heard the statistics: around 90 per cent of women who lose weight regain it — often plus some. If we break it down further, women who lose a significant amount of weight (through non-surgical means) will regain a third of it within a year and all of it within five years. That's enough to strike fear into our hearts. And as if that wasn't enough, we get even more scared when we consider our own frailties, weaknesses, past mistakes and how easily we succumb to even the tiniest temptation. Over and over again. Living in fear is not only sad. It almost guarantees we won't succeed.

A woman who wants to lose weight almost always follows this pattern: she sets physical goals, then changes her behaviour in ways that will help her achieve them. But she forgets about the other major player in the game: her mind. Big mistake. Even when she has lost weight, she's living with a savage psychological fear of regaining weight. Eventually that fear wins out. If she was confident instead of fearful, the weight would stay off permanently. It's literally that straightforward (as long as she didn't toss away all her good habits). It's like poor people who win the lottery. Most of them are back where they started financially within a year or two of banking the money. Sure, at first they go crazy buying stuff, but they don't do it with confidence; they do it like a pauper. They're thinking and behaving like a poor person who lives in fear that the money will all dry up. So it does. The sad truth is that rich people are much better equipped to win lotto because they can handle it psychologically, just as thin people would be so much better at losing weight and keeping it off. But that's just not fair, is it?

Check out this list. When women regain weight they believe it is because they have slipped up in their eating and activity behaviours. This is certainly true, but what they really need to think about are the reasons driving this change in behaviours — because these are psychological:

→ Inability to accept that their goal is unrealistic for their body, so struggling to maintain extreme diets and exercise regimes.

→ Being stuck on a 'number' as their only marker of weight-loss success, especially when the number they try to get down to is way too small and therefore too difficult to achieve.

→ Failure to perceive modest weight loss as a triumph, so denial of deserved pleasure.

→ Losing incentive because of lack of support, encouragement and praise.

→ Being stuck in other areas of life, fuelling boredom, misery, sadness and disappointment, which, in turn, fuels weight gain.

Consider these quotes from women who've lost significant amounts of weight:

As soon as I achieved my goal weight I didn't know what to do. My whole life didn't seem to have any meaning, I had no purpose. I just hit the fridge.

I was only 3kg from my goal weight. I kept thinking that one piece of chocolate couldn't hurt. And of course it wouldn't . . . if I had one piece then didn't have another for a week or more. But my mind wouldn't play that game. It told me, 'Oh well, I've had one now, I might as well have another. I can get back on this diet thing tomorrow.' And I did for a day or two but my resolve had cracked. I was back on the treadmill. I was gone.

I felt like I wasn't trained to handle my new weight. I knew I looked good on the outside — but inside I was shipwrecked, terrified. I knew that my new happiness was tenuous. That my whole world could collapse if I put on a single kilo. So then I started to obsess about food and from that moment I knew it was over.

For me it was a case of sneaking just a bit more food. Come on, I'd been dieting for a year; surely I deserved a little treat? I put on a kilo, then another, and before I knew it all my new clothes were pinching around my stomach and I couldn't get my new pants done up . . . the weight came back faster than it left in the first place.

So what's success?

Success is such an individual thing in weight loss. Even the experts can't agree: they avoid giving a definitive answer to what equals success, mostly I think because they don't want to make fools of themselves. We all know that lots and lots of diets can claim short-term success — even the strange and potentially damaging ones. But not many go the distance. And you know what? That's generally not the diet's fault, although some diets are unsustainable over time. It's not even the fault of the woman on the diet. It's just that you haven't programmed yourself — by that I mean your thinking and/or behaviour — for long-term success. So pause and consider what weight-loss success would be for you, because if you can't define what you want you won't recognise it when you get there.

What's your idea of weight-loss success?
- → Is it the moment you hand over the cash for your new size (insert your ideal size here) jeans?
- → Is it the first compliment you receive when you step out in them?
- → Is it at the point when you've kept the weight off for six months? A year? Five years?
- → Is it being free of dieting and all the weight-related guilt and disappointment?
- → Is it being able to walk past the pantry knowing it's full of chocolate biscuits?
- → Is it being so interested in your own life that you forget the biscuits are even there?

Going the distance

This is something that you need, and deserve, to know: lasting weight loss is a two-tier project. Your success depends on paying equal attention to both phases:

1.   Weight loss
2.   Weight maintenance

So the idea is that you lose weight to get within your ideal range (phase one), then you forget about losing more weight and do what needs to be done to keep yourself there (phase two). Put like that it sounds simple — but it's not. The problem (and it's a very big problem) is that most women stay forever in the weight-loss phase because even when they've lost a lot of weight they just want to drop a little more — so they never advance to the weight-maintenance phase. To be fair, they're mostly not aware of the importance of separating the two stages. Most diets are all about helping you lose weight — and that's what traps you in the 'trying to lose' cycle. Weight-loss programmes, like diets, make most of their money out of people 'trying to' achieve their goals, not those who have already done it. The better programmes devote equal attention to weight loss and weight maintenance. Beware of those that don't mention maintenance — or they've just tacked it on the end of their weight-loss method as an afterthought.

You probably think I'm doing the same thing because, after all, this is chapter 11 and our work is close to done. But I'll defend myself by saying that many of the ideas you've read so far contribute to helping you keep weight off — as well as losing it. For example, you simply can't expect to keep weight off without strategies for dealing with stress, understanding why you 'comfort eat' and changing your relationship with food. However, it's important to devote a specific section to weight-loss maintenance because it's where so many of our best efforts to lose weight fall apart. So here it is . . .

Keeping weight off after slaving to lose it

Let me tell you another secret. Actually, it's not a secret. You already know this secret, it's just that you don't want to admit it. Me neither, really. None of us do. It's this: **women love the whole dieting thing**. It makes us feel like we're taking charge. It gives us something to do. It's 'a project'. When we're messing around with our eating and exercise levels we're achieving. If we're losing weight then we're getting praise. All of which is why we feel so great when it's working — and so distraught and empty when it's not. And why, when we get to our goal weight, we get all messed up and start piling it on again.

Diet gurus mainly ignore the weight-maintenance stage because it's not as sexy or exciting as weight loss. In other words, it won't make them any money. But this is a very stupid and very mean approach. It's stupid because sound weight maintenance stops us from ballooning out to bigger than we were in the beginning. And it's mean because ballooning out is exactly what happens when we keep battling to lose weight instead of switching into maintenance mode. It's also a sneaky trick because (and you may not want to hear this) dieting is the easy part of weight loss because it is generally **very structured**. As soon as you take the structure away, everything often starts to fall apart.

For women trapped in the weight-loss phase, the intense and often life-long focus on losing weight is the root of so much dissatisfaction. Truly. How many of us, even when we've lost weight, are fully satisfied with what we've done? We're usually just a kilo or two from our mental target so we **keep trying**. Or we're so freaked out about the potential to regain the weight that we can't relax and enjoy what we've achieved.

Weight-loss success stories would have us believe that it's possible to achieve the impossible. That we can carve a third, or even half, off our body weight and happily maintain it. But research tells most of us (and remember that I'm not talking about women who are morbidly obese here) that it's very, very difficult to sustain weight losses of more than 10–15 per cent of your initial body weight. Most women don't know that. Even those who do know it have a very hard time accepting it. But being realistic about your goal weight is important because it underpins your ability to accept your weight and, ultimately, yourself.

So what's realistic?

Your body has a place (in terms of weight, size, muscle and fat) at which it is most comfortable **and** functions at its best. If you are healthy, that's where it will settle whether you give it permission or not. It's better to think of this as an ideal 'range' of several kilograms rather than a specific point. Your ideal weight range is that which is most realistic for you; the place at which your weight is compatible with your height, bone mass and body composition. It's the weight at which you can function or perform at your best. It's the weight at which you look great, according to everyone else. And it's the weight at which you're just a few kilos too heavy, according to yourself. (Your mind sets that slightly too-hard goal in order to drive you insane, remember.)

I bet you could identify your body's ideal range without too much trouble. I bet you've been there, probably more than once. It's the place at which your best efforts at weight loss slow down and it becomes very, very tough to drop any more. As long as you've put in a fairly consistent effort over time, that's the time you should STOP trying to lose weight and start thinking about staying where you are. Most women don't though; their minds instruct them to lose just a little, teeny weeny, bit more. And it's that desire that closes around them like a steel trap and fuels ongoing dissatisfaction with their body. It also keeps them restricting their food intake to such an extent that they inevitably give up.

Your aim is to find your body's ideal weight range. Allow yourself around 5kg fluctuation so that you don't freak out every time you gain 1kg. You are being way too tough if you don't allow your body to have natural day-to-day and week-to-week fluctuations because that's part of being female. Wouldn't you love to package up your hormones and give them away sometimes? Preferably to a man. But back to the story . . .

Your ideal weight range is the place at which you will look your most gorgeous (provided you have halfway decent taste in clothes) AND you will feel strong and energetic AND you will be able to stay that way with very little effort. It's the constant quest to do just a little better that keeps us miserable. And I'm not just talking about weight loss, either. I'm talking about all aspects of our lives. How many people do you know that can't help wanting what their friends, neighbours and family have? How many times have you felt that tinge of envy yourself? It's human but it's not helpful. We should all save our envy for the people who are satisfied with what they have — even if it's not much — because they at least have a shot at happiness.

So how long will it take?

Women always want to know how long it will take for their weight to settle. No one can answer this absolutely because it depends on a woman's unique combination of the many factors we've discussed: genetics, biology, weight-loss history, environment, stress and happiness levels, eating and activity habits, and your approach to weight loss (this time around). But if I was forced to be generic about it, I'd say your weight should settle between six months and a year after you've been making a consistent effort to reduce it. It may take longer, of course, if you genuinely have a very large amount of weight to lose.

The key is to **stop** trying to lose weight when you reach this point because it's not compatible with what you need to do to maintain your new stable weight. You want to relax your efforts to restrict food a little, but not abandon them.

To do that you need to develop, practise and establish weight-maintenance skills that will enable you to:

→ Accept the possible rather than chase the impossible.
→ Understand why your weight fluctuates (and therefore not panic about it).
→ Maintain your weight when others have lost interest and you're not getting praise and encouragement.
→ Lose the notion of a timeframe for weight loss — so your good habits and good thinking stay with you.
→ Learn to deal with setbacks.
→ Identify your own 'risk' factors and know how to respond to them.
→ Know that your weight won't change without the protection of a 'diet' or 'plan'.
→ See weight maintenance as part of your life instead of a major goal.

When you've got all that sitting in your head, you can forget about your weight altogether. Well, as much as a woman ever could.

About two years ago I went on yet another diet and lost 12kg.
I was 94kg and my aim was to get down to 75kg, because that's been
my aim for the past 15 years! This time I got down to 82kg, gave
up, bought some new funky clothes, and when I put them on it just
occurred to me that I looked quite good. Since then I've come to
see myself as an 80–85kg woman. If I walk the dog every day and
don't go too crazy with food I can stay here. It's been a year now and
I realised the other day that I'd lost that panicky feeling about food
and eating and my weight. It's still there a little bit but I don't feel so
trapped. In fact, I feel kind of free.
Fiona, 42

Dear Free-ona,
I don't really need to write back to you do I? Come work with me
and help spread the word. You've conquered your head and let your
body do the rest. Well done; 80–85kg women rock the world. But
only if they believe they can.

Doing things differently

Psychologists go on and on about the importance of change. That's because we assume, when people come to see us, that they want their lives to be different; in other words, better, easier, more fun, more meaningful. But while wanting change is a valid goal we have to be careful about the size of the change that we're aiming for — and the pace at which we go after it. People are built differently mentally, as well as physically, so it's important that any goals and strategies are designed to suit the individual — not the psychologist. 'Change' can be a scary word, too, so the best plan is generally just to encourage people to start doing things a little differently in terms of both their thinking and behaviour.

Changing your behaviour

Changing your food-related behaviour is obviously essential to achieving lasting weight loss and we've already covered lots of ways to do this. But because it is actually easier to lose weight than maintain your new weight it's important to:

Transition properly from whatever weight-loss plan you've been using so that you don't just 'stop' your diet and go back to whatever you were doing before. The most tragic weight-loss stories come from women who've put in the hard yards for months, lost weight, looked amazing then gradually returned to all their old patterns (and been doubly depressed because of it). Please don't do that. Hold on to your gains: you deserve it.

Use guidelines to govern your eating and activity from this point on. This is essential to achieving lasting weight loss and, if you don't have these, then you are wasting your time from the outset. Over time, you may have come up with some rules for yourself and, if so, I'm urging you to write them down, keep them where you can see them until they're stamped into your psyche, and start to follow them. If you need some help, I've included my list at the end of this chapter. Some of you will have taken a sneak preview way back when I first mentioned these guidelines. These are based on the best ideas of all the women I've seen, heard or read about. So even if you're still not sure about me, you can trust them.

Reprogramming your mind

Headings like this always spook me. They make me think of cult-centred brainwashing techniques, chanting affirmations or surgical fiddling with your neural hardwiring (through a hole bored in your skull). Which probably just tells me I need to put the horror novels away, especially late at night. Reprogramming your mind is simply training yourself to think in a different way. Habitually. It is a matter of learning to think more about the things that are helpful and less about those that are not. Of course this is done by small degrees. You don't wake up one morning and leap out of bed with a whole new set of thoughts. It takes time.

If you have lost weight, even a little bit, these are the most important things to think about. Notice that each of these points is directed at YOU. That's the key. There is no such thing as a generic strategy for success or one-size-fits-all plan for weight loss. You have to adopt a way of thinking that is specific to yourself. And these are the key steps in achieving that:

- → Accepting **yourself** and your weight.
- → Identifying what has worked **for you.**
- → Focusing on the benefits of weight loss **to you.**
- → Acting 'as if' you've already succeeded.

When enough is enough (or accepting your weight before you're quite ready)

The whole point of this weight-loss book is to get you thinking less about your body and food and more about you and your life. In an ideal world I'd love us all to hug ourselves, eat food only when and where required, and get on with the business of living. But I'm a realist. I know women want to **lose** weight. We don't just want to take what we've got and be happy with it. That's all very well if you are already thin. But most of us, well, we're not happy with what we've got. Worse, we're always on the alert for a left-field attack from some malicious fat cells. We want to weigh **less** than we do now — not the same. This is called being female in the twenty-first century.

But this is what I want to say: you don't even have to get to within your ideal weight range to feel better about yourself or to claim success. Even modest weight loss will make you feel good. Even the feel of slightly looser jeans, even being able to squeeze a finger between your stomach and your waistband brings a small burst of pleasure. Right? **So aim small.** Or at least don't aim so big. Set little goals. And when you feel some success, even minuscule, allow yourself to see it as an achievement. Achieving an easy goal is better for you psychologically than not achieving a hard one. And if it's too easy you can always come up with another goal later on.

I accept that **aiming small** is a challenging idea. If, like Fiona, you've had a specific number in your head for a long time then it's not easy to let it go and accept another number — especially a bigger one. It always worries me when women tell me they want to lose 25kg or 30kg (or more). Usually they say this just after they've (re)joined a gym and are pumped for success. Maybe they do need to lose this much, and maybe they will, but setting a numerical goal of Mount Everest proportions is making it unnecessarily hard and tipping the odds sharply towards failure. If they would just think about how they'd like to look and what they'd like to wear they'd be far more likely to succeed — and get there far sooner. As I've said before, weight loss is not a numbers game. If you are still thinking that way as this book nears a close then you've got a problem. Actually, no, I have. I've spent months writing this book and I still haven't made my message clear. Sigh. If I hadn't said all those things about the dangers of comfort eating I'd be running in the general direction of my fridge.

So . . . please, stay away from the numbers. If you've lost a little weight — or next time you lose some — pull out that picture you created way back in chapter 2 of your ideal, but very realistic, self. Then ask yourself this question:

How close am I to looking like this?

If it seems like a long way off, show the picture to three friends and ask them if they think it's possible for you to ever look like this. If the answer is 'no' from all three, then maybe you need to make yourself a new picture. If only one says 'no', consider whether you really need her as a friend. And go hug the other two. And if you are already in the ballpark, give or take a new outfit or some better fashion advice, then it's time to stop trying to lose weight and start teaching yourself to be happy with what you've got.

Note: I'm serious about the importance of clothes. What you wear can make an enormous difference to the way you look and your perception of the way you look. So if you can't trust your sisters or your friends, think about investing in some fashion advice because why not look as good as you can. It's a way better treat to give yourself than chocolate.

Getting happy with your body (and other foreign ideas)

This is one of the bizarre things about weight loss. All the public talk, the glossy magazines and weight-loss literature, focus on success: the women who've MADE IT, the women who will have better lives because they weigh less. But this is not an accurate reflection of what women are thinking. Not even close. What women really think about is 'failure'. We're thinking that we don't have the strength or the willpower to lose weight; we're thinking that even trying is futile; we're thinking that we're useless and **fat**. And even when we've done well, and lost a few kilos, we're thinking that it's not enough — or we're living in fear of the slightest weight gain.

So I don't want us to think any more about what's gone wrong. We've done enough of that — and we're very, very good at it. Instead, I want us to think about what's gone right.

Women's efforts at weight loss are littered with success. Really they are. It's just that we never allow ourselves to think about what we did right because we're too busy concentrating on our 'failures' and our fears — and working up the energy and resolve to try all over again. Mostly where it all goes wrong is that we fail to notice, and therefore accept, that we've done well. We fail to notice **why** we've done well. We fail to capture our success.

STUFF TO DO: **WHAT WORKS FOR ME**

Return again to your past efforts to lose weight. Go back to those you identified right back at the start if you need to. Pick your best one. Come on. Even if you're still depressed by the whole weight-loss thing, I bet you've had some success at some time. That's why you're still in the game: you actually know you can do it. You actually have a plan that works. It just hasn't worked over time.

Now, complete the diagram over the page. In the middle write down the name of the plan that has worked best for you or just describe it in a way that is meaningful for you. In all the spaces outside this, write down all the reasons it worked for you at that time. So maybe you made time to get to the gym four times a week, you had a friend that went with you and was supporting your efforts to lose weight, you halved the amount of food you ate, you cut snacks and so on.

Consider all the different types of factors. Here are a few examples:

Environment — supportive people (name them); shopping habits; when and how you buy food; amount and type of food in your house; cooking facilities/who cooks; proximity of takeaway outlets; going to weight-loss group weekly.

Behaviour — eating regularly; cooking well; getting up in time for breakfast; sitting down to eat; monitoring your portions; not eating in front of the TV; replacing trips to the snack box at work with trips to the water cooler; exercise/activities (be specific); cutting out the pasta; reducing to one slice of bread a day.

Psychological — having a plan for when feeling stressed out; meaningful activities to counter boredom; being fulfilled at work/home and in relationships; making time for myself; celebrating my success (but not with food); feeling good about myself and my efforts.

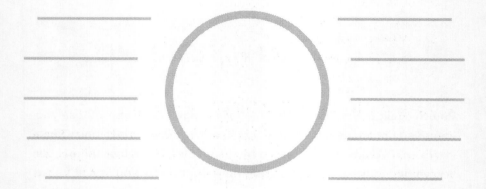

If you get stuck filling in the spaces, think about the major obstacles to you losing weight or what has eventually tripped you up, and how you countered them. Because if, at any time, you have been able to lose weight, you have been doing something right. The idea is to identify and reproduce the strategies that worked for you.

Benefits of weight loss to YOU

Listing the benefits of weight loss might seem boring to you. But it's important to embed this deep into your psyche because it will start to direct your behaviour. And, at the very least, it prevents you from dwelling on the downside of not losing weight. Here are some examples, but it's important that you create a list that is meaningful to you. Phrase it in language that suggests you are already at your ideal weight, therefore already getting these benefits. Here are some of the more common ones women offer, which might match yours, but make your list unique. Try to think about what might make your list different from your sister's or your friend's:

→   I look better.
→   I'm able to buy and enjoy a wider range of clothes.
→   I'm fitter/stronger so I have more energy for . . . .
→   I'm healthy.
→   I look acceptable in a swimsuit or in gym gear.
→   I'm can enjoy wearing summer clothes.
→   I have more respect for myself.
→   I feel more vibrant.
→   My skin looks better.
→   I'm more confident which for me means . . . .

Acting 'as if', or fake it till you make it

I would have found a way to put this in any book I wrote because I love it. It works. Really. Not just in weight loss — but in any area of your life (except sex because faking it should be about making yourself feel good not someone else). But here's the truth: the more you are able to align yourself with who/what you want to be, the closer you are to it actually happening. So the more you act like the relaxed, confident (well-dressed) woman you imagined yourself way back at the start of the book, the more you will look — and feel — like her. And please, don't just be this woman for the sake of your weight. Be her for the sake of your life. The payback will be heftier than any weight you imagined yourself to be.

Dealing with setbacks

I wish I could say that once you lose weight and set about maintaining it, you will never again have a problem. But if I said that you would snap this book shut and call me ignorant. And you would have a very good point. We are people. And the fascinating, heart-warming thing about people is that we stuff up. We sometimes do the wrong things, with the wrong people, in the wrong places, at the wrong times. And that includes what we do with food and activity. Sometimes we'll fall over. That's okay. As long as we get up again and stay in the game. If you get up one more time than you fall over then you are winning. The only real failure is giving up altogether.

The first thing to do when there's a problem is to recognise and acknowledge it. Most women who start to gain a little weight go into psychological denial. Sure, there's a slight tremor, a shudder of panic, but they manage to sidestep it as they increase their pace en route to the vending machine. This is how to anticipate, accept and respond to a problem:

1 **Define your (realistic) ideal weight range.** Be easy on yourself and try to see the bigger picture (a few kilos will not make any difference to the quality of your life).

2 **Monitor your weight gain in a way that works for you.** Is it the shrinking waistband of a favourite pair of jeans? Is it the tendency of the excess to keep shaking even after you've come to a stop? Do you like to weigh yourself once a month? Is your increase a gradual trend or a sudden leap? Be honest: if your weight really is back on the uphill climb then accept that you need to do something about it.

3 **Identify the specific cause.** So if it's stress that is causing you to overeat or binge, what is the precise reason for the stress? And what can you do about it?

4 **Plan a (rational) response.** So maybe pull out your food/ activity guidelines and make sure you are following them. Then maybe sit down and identify what's changed in your life lately — and what you could do about it? (Tip: don't just promise yourself that you'll eat nothing the next day and go for an exhausting run. Because that's a knee-jerk response that you won't be able to sustain . . . so you're wasting your time — again.)

5 **Do it.** Act on the response you've planned above. Even if the thing you do is really, really tiny like cutting out the brownie you've started to have at morning tea. Then do it again the next day. It will put you back in charge of your body.

6 **Re-read the appropriate chapter of this book.** Sometimes we just need a reminder to set our behaviour and our thinking back on track. And you might as well get your money's worth.

Your personal weight-maintenance plan

Drawing up a personal weight-maintenance plan can be useful because it helps you consolidate everything you've come to know about you and your weight. I'm not going to ask you to make a big deal of this because it goes against the very philosophy that I've been trying to impart. That is, to keep you from thinking — day and night — about your body and your weight. However, it is important to have a really good grasp of why you want to stay at a particular weight (the benefits), of all the ways that help you to do this and of your vulnerabilities/warning signs. And, most of all, how you can best respond to risk.

Your vulnerabilities

How do you get into trouble? I'm not just talking about your weight. I'm talking more generally. Are you vulnerable to particular people, environments or events? Is it your impulsivity? Your neediness? Your loneliness? Are you highly sensitive to criticism? Do you get angry quickly? Or overwhelmed by stress?

You might wonder what all this has to do with your weight. Actually, I bet by now you won't be wondering that at all. You'll know that the kind of person you are: your biology and history, the way you think, behave and react has everything to do with your weight. Just as we all have strengths, we all have trigger points and vulnerabilities. And it's important to have a good understanding of them in relation to food and activity.

So ask yourself these questions. But **don't** write down your answers because this is not what we want to reinforce psychologically. We'll get to that in a minute:

- → Which environments are most risky for me?
- → Which situations/activities cause me to change my helpful eating/activity? Or place me at risk of doing so?
- → Which moods or emotions are most risky for me?
- → Who are the people who are most likely to wreck my good intentions?
- → Is there a pattern to my poor eating or becoming sedentary?

Answering these questions will help you keep track of your most vulnerable times. And to develop and deploy strategies to counter them, many of which we've explored throughout this book.

Remember . . .

Replacing unhelpful thinking and behaviour works better than trying to eradicate it. Now, reverse these questions AND write down your answers. These are the things that will help. And these are the ones we need to reinforce.

My plan

Which environments encourage my best eating/activity behaviours?	
Which emotions are most helpful in encouraging good habits and how can I create more of them?	
Which people are most helpful and how can I copy them/see more of them?	

What's going on in my life when I eat well and take regular activity?	
Is there a pattern to my helpful eating/ activity behaviours and how can I replicate it?	
When I start to slip, how do I respond? Immediately? Longer term?	

Your answers are the foundation of your weight-maintenance plan. That's why I really, really want you to write them down. So please don't cheat. Then, whenever things get a bit tough, you can pull this plan out to remind yourself what works for YOU.

The penultimate food for thought

If you are trying to lose weight then you will stuff up.

Think small. Set little goals. Aim to achieve the possible — not chase the impossible.

Focus on what you've done right in weight loss — not what you've done wrong.

Fake it till you make it (but not with sex).

Big, fit women can rock the world. But only if they believe they can.

Weight-loss success is being so happy that you forget there are biscuits in the tin. Ahhh, if only.

The ultimate food for thought: THE RULES

These are not really rules because I don't want you to think I'm telling you what to do. Even if I am. Let's call them guidelines for helping you lose weight then maintain that loss that I **totally** expect you to comply with (unless you have an utterly brilliant excuse).

Eating and weight

→ Eat breakfast (every day, even when you don't feel like it). Eat it early. If you are sitting down to breakfast at 9.30am on a weekday then you are asking for trouble.

→ Try to keep meal times consistent.

→ It's okay to skip a meal, just not breakfast.

→ Only eat when you are hungry, but don't wait till you're ravenous.

→ You don't have to lick the plate clean. You don't have to eat food you don't like.

→ One carbohydrate group per meal only (i.e. no pasta and bread together. Or potatoes and bread). And keep the portions down.

→ Limit your bread intake. And that means slices, not loaves.

→ Sometimes you don't need any carbs in your meal.

→ Avoid fast food as often as you can and the same for processed and artificial foods.

→ Try not to eat too late in the evening. Especially try not to eat a heavy meal late in the evening. But, if you do, move around a bit before bed. However, keeping your intake down over 24 hours and being active are more important than making sure you have a light, early dinner.

→ Eat slowly. Aim to finish last.

→ Reduce your portions where possible. Most of us could eat less and still have had plenty.

→ Having morning and afternoon tea is a really dumb habit. Distract yourself.

→ Try not to snack between meals — you don't need them. Or if you must snack, make it small and healthy. (Yoghurt-dipped muesli bars are out.)

→ No second helpings. When you're tempted, wait. The moment will pass.

→ No desserts (okay that's a bit harsh, but save them for special occasions).

→ Cake is only for family birthday parties, except if you have 12 kids.

→ Think of food as food. Or fuel. Not a treat. Not a reward. Not a punishment. If you want a treat buy a magazine. Or lock the door and take a bath.

→ Don't weigh yourself. Or at least don't do it often.

Fluids

→ Drink water. It will keep you hydrated, it's calorie free and it helps purify the body. But you don't have to drink eight litres a day unless you enjoy spending a large amount of time in the bathroom.

→ A glass of wine is okay. Even two (this is my book, remember).

→ Beer will not contribute to your weight-loss efforts. Sadly.

→ A nip of spirits in itself won't hurt but what you put with it might.

→ Soft drinks or fizz are not good for your body. Phase them out.

→ Juice, other than the purest of the pure, isn't brilliant either. But it can taste so good that a little won't hurt.

→ Coffee and tea. Well, I wouldn't give these up altogether so I can't ask you to. But one decent coffee a day is enough. And train yourself not to buy a little something to have with it.

→ Sports drinks? Only if you are an elite athlete. Sorry.

Physical activity

→ Physical activity **after** eating is better than the other way around, although I concede that it's hard to do breakfast first if you get up at dawn to work out. Just don't hit the bacon and eggs after you've done it. (Maybe occasionally.)

→   Don't make a big deal of planning your food intake before and after physical activity. Just go with what you need.

→   Being active, or walking, after the evening meal is smart. Going to bed on a full stomach is not.

→   Go to the park. Take the stairs. Move at every chance you get.

→   Walk daily. Then start to walk faster.

→   Thirty minutes or more physical activity five days a week is your goal. Aerobic — heart pumping, puffing, sweating — is best but anything is good.

→   Look for ways to get your heart rate up as often as possible. Sex counts if you make an effort.

→   Five minutes' physical activity every day is the minimum and better than nothing. But only just.

And that's all you have to do for the rest of your life. So commit these ideas to memory and then forget about them. Trust your mind and your body to do the rest.

12 MY BUM LOOKS BRILLIANT AFTER ALL

'You have got to discover you, what you do, and trust it.' *Barbra Streisand, legend of screen and microphone*

So that's it. You've read the book, done the activities, taken on some new ideas and started to think and behave differently. And even if you haven't yet put it all into action, you have a plan and some strategies in your head: you know what you need to do. Up until now, we've kept on the weight trail and related topics, which was the whole point and why you read the book. But now it's time to step back and think a little beyond your body, to ponder the bigger questions, because while your goal at the outset was to downsize your body, mine was always to supersize your life.

Are you happy?

When I was a kid I was fascinated by the folklore myth that suggested there was a pot of gold at the end of every rainbow. I believed it — and I wanted it. So when I was about 10 and a vivid rainbow appeared one afternoon I grabbed a backpack (I suspect with nothing in it except for underwear) and went hunting for the gold. For what seemed like hours I scrambled towards the point where the rainbow appeared to hit the ground. Of course I never even got close; the rainbow kept darting out of my reach until, eventually, it disappeared. It occurred to me then, as I sat there on the hill with my pack full of things I couldn't eat, that getting what I wanted from life might be harder than I thought. And also that the happy endings in fairy stories might actually be a crock of, well, the proverbial (insert your favourite swearword here).

Everyone, repeat everyone, wants to be happy. For most people, happiness is conditional on a change in their circumstances. So they see happiness not as something they have right now, but as something they'll get when they, for example, have more money; change jobs or the boss leaves; find a partner; have a baby or — you guessed it — lose weight. Not surprisingly, happiness remains as elusive as the rainbow's pot of gold despite the frenzied attention it has had in recent years. In the Western world, thousands of books on happiness are published each year, at least 100 universities offer happiness courses and the entire life-coaching industry is built on the promise of bliss. This is kind of ironic at a time when our depression and anxiety statistics are at an all-time high — and rising. Interestingly, too, research tells us that Western world dwellers don't have a monopoly on the good life: as much joy abounds in impoverished Nigeria as in New York City. And right behind Nigeria as the world's 'happiest countries' come Mexico, Venezuela and El Salvador, according to a world values survey carried out at the University of Michigan. So where are the affluent countries? The very fact that multimillion-dollar incomes, Fifth Avenue penthouses and designer shoes are not direct correlates of happiness is a vote in favour of a simpler life with good relationships, meaningful ways of passing the time and a few laughs as the basis of true fulfilment.

Research and literature summarise the key psychological attributes of happy people as follows. They're in no particular order:

→   Optimism.
→   Good self-esteem.
→   Supportive (and fun) close relationships.
→   Appreciation for what you have.
→   Sense of progress or achievement.
→   Sense that you are in charge of your own life.

→ Involvement in meaningful/absorbing work or interests.

→ Behaving in accordance with your values.

Which of them could you give a tick to? Which could you improve on? It's worth thinking about because improvements in one or more of these areas can radically change your satisfaction with life.

A human hierarchy of wants

Historically, human happiness was founded on survival; people focused on what they needed, not what they wanted. American psychologist Abraham Maslow's post-World War II Hierarchy of Needs perhaps best illustrated this. Using a pyramid he explained how humans first sought to have their physiological needs met (air, water, food and sleep), then safety (security and stability), social (belonging, love and acceptance) and, finally, self-esteem and personal fulfilment. People who achieved the highest status were said to be self-actualised; that is, they had more peak experiences than everyone else and were more on track to becoming all they were capable of being. At the time it was groundbreaking stuff, but I bet if Maslow was alive now he would be astonished at our twenty-first century spin on his model. Now we take what we need for granted and spend our lives chasing down what we want. Being self-actualised is more likely to be about winning a place on America's Next Top Model (Down Under) or slipping into size-10 jeans when you've spent a lifetime straining the zip on a size 14.

During wartime and the depressions, it was a bit of a treat to be alive at the end of each day. People mattered. Shelter from the elements mattered. Food that wouldn't give you scurvy mattered. What did not matter was the presence in your lounge of a 50-inch high-definition flat-screen television or being able to carry 1000s of songs on an electronic device the size of your fingernail. And when it came to physical appearance, it was good enough to have a body that could breathe and move — in that order. Now we want it in the right proportions, cellulite- and wrinkle-free, tanned, buffed, polished and accessorised with all the right stuff. And when it's not, it's the font of so much misery.

Or is it?

Just for a moment, forget about your weight and think about your life. Don't just think about your work either. Ask yourself the following questions. There's no need to write down your answers but force yourself to answer them in your head, because that will put you way ahead of most people. The truth is that very, very few people can quantify what makes them happy. And the well-documented truth is that if you don't know what you want from life then you are highly unlikely to get it (even if you work really, really hard):

→ What makes you happy?
→ What makes you feel relaxed and content?
→ Who do you most like to be with? Do you spend enough time with them?
→ What do you love doing? What makes your heart thump?
→ What do you do without looking at the clock?
→ What's your idea of a perfect day?
→ Is your work or favourite interest meaningful? Why or why not?
→ What are you good at? What have other people complimented you on now and in the past? (Anything to do with your body doesn't count.)
→ What is your main contribution to the world?
→ If your life ended tomorrow would you be content with what you've done? Why or why not?

Think about your answers. Maybe you found them easy. If you struggled with your answers that's no big deal: many people do. But they are worth thinking about, and trying to quantify, because your answers and the way you act on them are the key to your satisfaction with life. Now try these questions (again, forget about your weight).

What are you looking forward to:

→ This week?
→ This month?
→ Within the next year?

- → In three years?
- → In five years?
- → How about 10?

That's the trap. Even when people know what makes them happy they often don't have a concept of how they can map that on to their current life and circumstances — now and in the future. If you find yourself answering 'no idea' to those questions then you need to have a serious chat with yourself. Because being oriented to, and excited by, your future is what fuels hope. And hope underpins happiness.

Passion, purpose and pleasure . . . or, three things that mess us up

Passion

Passion is just as hot as happiness in the self-help stakes, which bothers me because the search for it makes many people desperately unhappy. The inference is that unless you have a grand passion, there's no point to your existence. A lot of people get hung up on trying to figure out what their passion is and, if they can't identify it, feel even more useless. And it will be even worse for our daughters because they have grown up thinking that having a 'passion' is as central to their existence as lip-gloss — and just as easy to obtain.

Think about it. Passion used to be the descriptor for great and abiding love. Now it's something you have to go find and engage in; it's **the** activity that is supposed to get you up early and keep you up late; the untapped secret to having a glorious life. **Find your passion and you will find yourself. Find your passion and you will have the key to the Great Door of Happiness.**

Blah. Passion can also get us into an awful lot of trouble. It can make us highly emotive, irrational, argumentative and, well, downright stupid at times. The truth about passion is this: it's not necessary to be so good at something, or so enraptured by it, that it will dictate the course of your life. Besides, who's got time to go out on a passion hunt these days? Certainly not me. If I've got time to go on a hunt for anything it's going to be shoes. What does passion look like anyway? I have no idea. All I do know is that it can't be found in a packet or a tin or a tub tucked inside the freezer.

Purpose

Why are you here? What's your purpose? Purpose is a more credible aim than passion because it doesn't give the impression that you have to be ecstatic with joy every time you do this 'thing', but the concept of needing a purpose or calling still makes life difficult. I have read many, many books and theories on this topic and they mostly don't come close to helping us figure out our purpose. They just make us feel bad because we don't have one. To be fair, though, purpose is a hard thing to work out. We are not born knowing exactly why we're here. We don't even recall how the trip went; nine or so months in we were just forced (by nature, a pair of forceps or some other medical intervention) to take it. Sometimes we're just here because of someone else's bloody mistake. Which is not a great way to sell you on your own importance to the universe. However, once we're here there should be some sort of obligation to make the most of it. I get that and I'm trying. Hopefully you are too.

Do you ever look at those people who seem to know what they are doing, why they are here, from day one? Women such as Mother Teresa, who appeared infused with goodness from an early age, and pioneering nurse Florence Nightingale, who said this of her divine calling: 'Since I was 24 there never was any vagueness in my plans or ideas as to what God's work was for me.'

I have often envied them, although I know I'm so far short of their league that I don't spend too much time on it. They were born on a mission — and they stayed on one. I know the historians will get all uptight about my next claim but I'm still going to make it: in many ways these legendary women had it easier than us. That's because they knew what they had to do. Their path was lit. Fairy lights guided them all along the way. They didn't have the choices we have, choices that make life so complicated and confusing. It's worth remembering that the Mother Teresas and Florence Nightingales among us are rare. Most of us just bump along the path, feeling our way in the dark, not really having a clue. Sure we may do some interesting work at times, meet some great people, go to some interesting places . . . but we are too busy doing these things to know if they're in true alignment with our soul. How do you figure it out? Surely it's not just a matter of lying in a hot bath and waiting till the answer swirls up out of the steam. Eureka! I know why I'm here! Now I can get out of the bath and go change the world. After I've gotten dressed.

Lots of young people are desperate to figure out their true purpose or calling because they believe this will be the point at which they can really start to live. They also think that if they don't find this great Reason for Being, they might as well resign themselves to a boring and unfulfilled life. Gee, no wonder depression statistics are going up. But I understand what they're saying. When I was younger I used to stand on a beach, stare at the horizon and ponder the meaning of life. Until I realised I was standing there alone and it was much more fun to give up the deep stuff and go find the party. Now there's even more pressure to get it right when you're young because while you're sitting around playing Socrates the student loan is going up.

Finding your purpose in life shouldn't be given so much credence or made to sound so complex. I mean, we're only talking about a reason to get up other than to pay the bills. Nothing more. Just something interesting to do. Or, better still, a whole lot of interesting things to do. Lots of women (actually let me be controversial here and say most women) hit their middle years in a state of flux. It's sort of like staring at the destinations board at the airport when you don't have a ticket. You're caught between dreaming about jumping on the next flight to Hawaii and knowing that in less than an hour you'll be home staring at the walls or making meat loaf. A little depressing, but THAT'S THE WAY IT IS. It's just that when that's the way it's been for day after day, year after year, the cracks start to show.

Is this you? Are you feeling a little fed up with the whole deal? Maybe you've been immersed in the relentless process of raising kids? Maybe you desperately want a child and haven't been able to find/pin down a man of sufficient quality to do it with? Maybe your relationship or career has gone belly up or you've just started to feel that there's something more you could do with your life? Maybe you have a nagging disappointment you just can't shake? It doesn't matter too much what the scenario is, the outcome is just the same. If your life feels directionless, dull and repetitive, or frenetically busy, this is what you need to know: you don't have to be fixated with a purpose to have a great life. You do need to make some changes though (see previous chapters). And you may have to be brave to do it.

Pleasure (and fun)

Pleasure refers to decadent pursuits and all the things that go with them. A lot of people say that the stuff of pleasure — expensive toys, the latest electronics and gadgets, designer clothes and jewellery, offshore holidays and the like — don't bring happiness. Who are they kidding? These must be people who've never had any toys. Pleasure can bring happiness **but only if** it is woven into a meaningful life. So if you have a full life, good relationships, enjoyable and challenging work or interests, then the hot candlelit bath you take at the end of the day or the cold glass of wine or the walk at dusk will make you feel happy. However, here's the difference. If these leisurely pursuits are the key events in your day, if these are the things you look forward to then they will bring you no pleasure. It will feel like just another boring day — no matter how warm the bath or chilled the wine.

One of the signs of being clinically depressed is not getting pleasure from any previously enjoyed activities. I'm always intrigued when I ask people what they do for fun and they stare blankly back — like they've forgotten what fun is or maybe they never knew. Both of which are very unhelpful to their psychological health. Having fun is essential. It's actually a pretty simple thing. And cheap. You just have to book in time to do something for yourself and, then (this is the harder bit) give in to it. There is fun to be had in the bleakest of situations. How do you think Nigerians do it? The key is to be open to it.

Meaning, gratitude and contribution . . . or, three things that help

Meaning

Meaning is a more useful term than purpose or passion because it acknowledges that leading a good life doesn't have to be about doing 'one big thing' maniacally or superbly well for your whole life. Perhaps it's just something you decide to give or offer? Perhaps it's holding true to your values? Perhaps it's just the way you choose to live? One of the early proponents of meaning was Austrian psychiatrist and Holocaust survivor Viktor Frankl, a Jew, who was able to find meaning in suffering while in the Nazi concentration camps in World War II. He believed that people had choices even in the most difficult of circumstances, that the last of the human freedoms was choosing to live your own life in your own way, and that a man, or a woman, always had power over that. I thought this was brilliant when I read it and I still do: if living my own way is the only thing I could ever achieve I'd be happy.

In my work I see people who are so depressed they can barely get out of bed. When you look at the landscape of their lives, it's not surprising. What have they got to get up for? A man who's just told them he doesn't want them? A job they hate? A drawer full of bills they can't pay? Kids who just keep yelling at them? Too many people in midlife go through their days blindly; at any age, actually. But midlife is often when you start to really care about it because suddenly there's not so much time left. Most people think true meaning lies in their work. Maybe it does; quite often it doesn't. Either way it's a mistake pinning happiness on work, a raise or promotion because, no matter how cool or competent you are, you can't consistently control it. At some point in your life you will be professionally hurt (because everyone is) and when it happens you better have your self-worth hooked to something other than your work — or have a darn fine safety net in place. And if you don't believe me check out the statistics on how many people die in the grey zone between retirement and starting the life they've been working for all of their lives. To date, these statistics have largely related to men. But with more women now spending their entire adult lives in the workforce, the female post-retirement mortality rate will go up. Watch this space.

Making life more meaningful
If you've been waiting around, or even searching, for a meaningful life to appear before you, forget it. I have never met a person who found fulfilment like that. So how? The quickest way to get things started is to ask yourself this question: **is what I'm doing now how I want to spend the next 20 years?** If the answer is no, you need to do more. Not think

more. Do more. You won't discover your true calling (or even anything) at home in bed thinking about it. You have to do something. Or, better still, lots of things. A new job? Retraining? Study? A night class or new hobby? Volunteer work? These may not be your things — but something is. So this is what you have to do: one thing, right now, to move yourself forward. Even if it's random. Even if it's outrageous. Even if it feels wrong. Pick up the phone. Go see an art show. Check out a new store. Walk around an area you don't know. Wear something different. Go to an exercise class. Visit a polytechnic or university. Notice that none of these are food related (and you know I've done that on purpose).

See what happens. Try something. Then try something else. And the answers will come. But you have to commit to this: one random act every week. One thing that takes you beyond the comfy zone you like to stay within. One thing that you haven't done before, or something you have done, but in a new capacity — something new, something different, something crazy. Even if it leads nowhere, your life will be a little more interesting for having made the effort. And if you do find something that is meaningful and enjoyable to you, you can do lots of it and see where it takes you.

Being grateful

We've already talked about the role that gratitude or appreciation has in boosting our self-esteem and happiness. Gratitude has its basis in prayer with most religions asking followers to regularly express gratitude for the things and people in their lives. Happiness scientists have taken up this mantra and suggest that people show their appreciation more formally through journals, daily lists and the like. This practice doesn't take long and it does work for or at least help your state of mind. However, I always feel a bit strange about writing daily lists of things I'm grateful for — even though there are a lot of them. I read somewhere once that if the only thing you said at the end of every day was thank you, that would be enough. I like that because it fits with the whole range of spiritual beliefs — not to mention the hectic pace of modern life. So if lists are not your thing, just say thanks at the end of each day. On a good day, you can add a bit more detail. And when you're really exhausted, you can mutter your thanks and you've still done your bit.

Your unique contribution

One of the great thrusts of self-help psychology is that you need to 'go after' or 'get' what you can from life. Ask for what you want and you'll receive it. Think about what you want to attract into your life and it will come. The concept has merit but in some ways it's a self-serving approach. When you are thinking about what you want to do with your life, it's better to frame it as what you can give or offer — rather than what you can get or take. What can you offer to your family, your community, the world (actually, if you are a woman your family is probably getting enough but you get my point)? What's your unique contribution? And even if it seems like a really small thing, congratulate yourself. Then go out and keep delivering it. If you can't think of anything you are contributing, then maybe you need to change the way you think about the things you do.

If you are not giving something back you are missing out on a major way of feeling good about yourself. But here's a warning. Don't give so much that it messes up other areas of your life. That won't help. In fact you will be left with a whole lot of very needy people who love and rely on you but not much in the way of proper friends. It's not worth it. So figure out who matters to you most and devote some time to making them feel like they matter. Remember, a small daily act of kindness (especially an unexpected one) will make you feel even better than the person you did it for. So it's worth the effort.

Living well

Good psychological health is not the absence of stress, anxiety or depression. It's definitely not about what you weigh. It's about living a full, enriched life. It's about living the width of your life as well as the length of it. It's about having good relationships, doing something that's meaningful to you and having fun. We've all heard the saying about no one lying on their deathbed saying I wish I'd spent more time at the office. No one will ever say I wish I'd eaten more Brussels sprouts and fewer French fries (unless they are 40 and dying of an obesity-related condition). They'd probably say I wish I'd had more laughs, more friends and more ice cream (within reason). I wish I'd taken more days off, flouted more rules, worn zanier clothes and been more stupid, more often. I wish I hadn't dusted and vacuumed so much (I'm never going to be guilty of that one). I wish I'd spent less time trying to check out my bum in the mirror and more time taking it out to have fun. I wish I'd stood still sometimes and allowed people to get to know the real me. Because the real me was worth knowing.

It's up to you

When I was 15 I read a book about living that changed my life. It doesn't much matter what the book was because we all have experiences like that and I don't want to bore and bias you with mine. But, for me, a light went on. I realised right then that the quality of my life would depend on the way I chose to view it, and to live it. I realised it was up to me. And, after all these years and all the things that have happened, I still believe it. Sure, life takes twists and turns, circumstances and events are sometimes beyond our control, there is sadness and disappointment. And. Sometimes. Life. Just. Sucks.

But there are also many moments of great joy, excitement, learning, fun and intrigue. The point is that if you want to be fulfilled, you have to open your eyes and recognise the good stuff when it bites you on your slightly overweight bum. If you need to make changes, you need to know which changes to make, and which things to leave alone. If you want to live a truly great life, **you** have to do something about it. Sit around and hope for luck if you must, but it could be a very long wait. And leave it to God if that is your way, but remember that He is a very busy guy. I suspect he'd welcome you taking a proactive approach. Remember, though, that whatever path you choose, **you** have chosen it. And if you can live with it, everyone else certainly can.

Breaking up and happy endings (optimism is important, remember)

So, here we are at the end. I always find saying goodbye to people tough. But it has to end because the psychologist's ultimate goal must always be the person's independent function. You and I both know that you are capable of losing weight, and living well, without me. So that's it, we're done. It's time for you to get up off my couch and go do it.

I wrote this book for women because I was sick of society telling us we had to be skinny to be brilliant. More importantly, I was sick of us, and our daughters, believing it. Hopefully the secret of lasting weight loss has revealed itself to you during the time we've spent together. But, just in case, I'll spell it out. I can't stand too much subtlety. When I was in my 20s I read Napoleon Hill's *Think and Grow Rich* book 10 or so times waiting for his hidden 'secret' of making millions to jump out of the pages and club me over the head. It never did. That's why I'm still working. Actually that's not why I'm working. I'm working because I like to. I'm working at my particular job because I like it. And I wrote this book because I thought it might help someone. More than one person, if I did a really good job. Sorry to disappoint if you were hoping for something more profound, but I'm just not that deep.

So here's the secret:
Sort out your life and your weight will follow (as long as you are not a complete glutton and stick to some basic rules — your own or mine as outlined in the previous chapter).

And this is the secret to the secret:

→ Identify and face your problems. Then do something about them.

→ Eat less and move more. And you must have a meaningful reason to do this. Like staying alive and healthy; or improving your confidence so you can live more fully.

→ Get absorbed in something bigger than your weight and looks — so you've got something else to do and something else to think about. Maybe it's your work? A hobby or interest? Making a contribution? (Note: don't just focus on your kids because they will grow up and leave — at least that's the plan.) It doesn't matter what activity you choose but you won't lose weight permanently without one.

Finally, I'm contractually bound to stick with the traditions of the other chapters and leave you with some food for thought. So here goes.

Food for thought

The secret to a good life can't be found in the fridge. So don't look there.

You are a person with a bum attached, not the other way around.

Work on yourself, not your weight.

Think about how you want your life to be and make a plan to get there.

Break the plan down. Act on it. One step at a time. One day at a time.

And even if you don't have a plan, go do something. Anything.

Do it now. Because tomorrow is like the pot of gold at the end of the rainbow. Alluring but a con job. And not worth waiting around for.

Do these things and you will have a brilliant life. Which is way more important than anything that happens with your bum. And if you see me around, come say hi and tell me how your life's going. Because I was always more interested in you than your bum. But you already knew that, didn't you?

Recipe section

Oh no, there's nothing here.

I put this section in because I know you expected it. My mum expected it. In fact, she is kind of horrified that I would write a book about weight loss without a selection of low-fat recipes to help you buy, cook and eat healthily. That's what most weight-loss books offer and so here is my recipe section: I didn't want you to think this book was a rip-off because I'd left it out.

The reason I didn't include any recipes was because there are already thousands of recipe books that can do this job better than me. I quite like cooking sometimes but I don't want to pretend that I'm really good at it. Also, I don't want to treat you like you are stupid. You don't need that kind of help from me. You already know what a healthy recipe is. That is, any recipe without too much crap in it. You don't need to spend time thinking about it, or your weekly grocery budget trying to create it. Just buy, cook and eat food *without the crap in it.*

PS: You do know what crap is, don't you?

Crap. *noun.* urban slang (as pertains to food only). Unacceptable; something of poor quality; rubbish food sought after excessive alcohol intake; descriptor for UK school dinners (see Jamie Oliver); fried; over-salted; over-oiled; fatty; processed; tasty (oh heck, I knew there was a catch).

Acknowledgements

The simple truth is that you can't write a book on your own. Well, you can, but it would probably remain a stack of paper in your underwear drawer. So I'm grateful to all those who helped me get from there to here:

→ Rebecca, Tracey, Jennifer and the team at Random House for their professionalism and for making the publishing process easy and fun. And for just trusting me to do the business.

→ Greek philosophers Aristotle, Plato and Socrates for first alerting me to the mind–body connection. And then to my teachers, colleagues and friends in physical education and psychology for helping me to pursue it, and for so much support and guidance along the way.

→ My clients, who continue to be my greatest teachers.

→ My parents, John and Mary, and my extended family, who remind me how lucky I am. Ditto my friends, old and new; young and old.

→ My daughters and harshest critics, Kate and Tess, for just jokin' around. And their friends who campaigned for (and deserve) a personal mention: EK, Maddie and Jordy.

→ And, finally, my personal edit team for keeping my words honest and my ego small: Kate, my friend, who carries her knowledge in all the right places; and Kev, my husband, just because.

Karen Nimmo
July 2009